latest edition 8/02

Bennett's

COSMETIC FORMULARY

COMPILED BY

Editorial Staff, Chemical Publishing Co., Inc.

CHEMICAL PUBLISHING CO., INC.

New York 1993

CHEMICAL PUBLISHING CO., INC.

Printed in the United States of America

CONTRIBUTORS

Amerchol Corp.	Edison, NJ
Croda Inc.	Edison, NJ
Gattefosse Corp.	St. Priest Cedex, France
W. R. Grace & Co.	Lexington, MA
McIntyre Group, Ltd.	Chicago, IL
Mona Industries, Inc.	Paterson, NJ
Frank B. Ross Co., Inc.	Jersey City, NJ
Sutton Laboratories, div. GAF Chemicals	Chatham ,NJ
Union Carbide Corp.	Danbury, CT
R.T. Vanderbilt Co.	New York, NY

TABLE OF CONTENTS

PREFACE

In 1990 we lost our oldest and most prestigious author and friend, Harry Bennett at age 95. He is sorely missed.

It was his wish that the "COSMETIC FORMULARY" continue with or without him. Our editorial staff has put together this volume, and shall continue to do so without making any changes in style or presentation.

We quote Harry Bennett from an earlier edition. "The purpose of this book is to correlate the most practical, up-to-date information and formulas in the cosmetic and allied fields. Since the knowledge in these fields is largely empirical, theories and opinions should be taken with the proverbial grain of salt. No two chemists or manufacturers will agree exactly on any formula. It is manifestly impossible to suit everyone. A formula is useful essentially as a starting point or as the source of an idea.

Although the manufacture of cosmetics in general is often an elaborate procedure, the technique is more manual than creative. Most cosmetic products can be prepared by the average person provided with a formula and common sense. If a procedure results in disappointment, it may be assumed that the trouble is due to improper technique, incorrect or impure quantities or materials, lack of knowledge of the specific properties of certain ingredients, or perhaps failure to realize that the product conforms only to specific and not to general requirements.

The creation of new formulas and new products is restricted, of course, to the specialist. Given a satisfactory formula, anyone can successfully produce a batch of cold cream, but to alter that cream, to modify its properties in conformity with certain desired ends, requires knowledge and experience. Although the whys and wherefores of cosmetic formulation were originally founded on tradition and based on rule-of-thumb experiments, with seemingly little rhyme or reason, the number of chemists employed in the cosmetics industry is steadily increasing. Cosmetics manufacturers are beginning to realize more and more the value of the chemist. Those who cannot engage a fulltime chemist are turning to with less tendency to deteriorate, and they are in a position to keep up with new developments.

Educational institutions, which in the past have paid little heed to this industry, are now aware of its importance. Many high schools are giving simple courses in making cosmetics in connection with their domestic science courses. Colleges, too, are awakening and preparing students to take their places in this tremendous industry.

It is hoped that this text will prove a starting point for education in the field of cosmetics manufacture. The editors will appreciate suggestions and criticisms from readers of this work with a view to extending its usefulness in further editions."

Grateful acknowledgment is made to the Contributors for their valuable suggestions and contributions.

CHEMICAL PUBLISHING CO., INC.

INTRODUCTION

Manufacturing Cosmetic Products

A major portion of cosmetic products can be manufactured by using relatively inexpensive laboratory equipment. Many formula procedures only require some combination of mixing, pulverizing, and heating. The chemist can therefore experiment with a variety of formulas without a substantial outlay of money.

It is always important to practice good housekeeping in the laboratory to keep the ingredients and the final product unadulterated. If the product requires a preservative, use an adequate amount so the cosmetic will not have too short a shelf life.

Choosing the appropriate package for the product is a practical consideration. The packaging should be based on the nature of the product itself. Where is it going to be used? If it is going to be carried in a handbag, or used at a dressing table, the container should possess some aesthetic qualities. If the product is highly perishable the container should incorporate the protective qualities that are essential to the product's maintenance.

Legal Considerations

In the United States, cosmetic manufacture and trade were brought under government regulation for the first time by the Federal Food, Drug, and Cosmetics Act of 1938, which today under the Federal Trade Commission and the Food and Drug Administration protects the consumer against the sale of adulterated, dangerous, or mislabeled cosmetics.

The Food and Drug Administration regulates the use of cosmetic pigments (organic and inorganic colorants). If an organic colorant is labeled D & C certified colorant, it can't be used in food or areas on or around the eyes. It can be used in lipstick, rouge, face powder, nail approved and listed by the Food and Drug Administration for cosmetic use, they can be included in all the cosmetic products already mentioned and also in eye preparations.

IMPORTANT

The use of FD & C Red No. 2 has been banned in some countries. Check for an appropriate legal substitute.

The information contained in this book is presented in good faith, and we believe it to be correct. However no warranty as to accuracy of results or fitness for a particular use is given, nor is freedom from patent infringement to be inferred except as expressly noted. It is offered solely for your consideration.

Chapter I

ANTIPERSPIRANTS AND DEODORANTS

Roll-On Antiperspirant

#1

A	VEEGUM HV	1.00
	Deionized Water	29.00
B	Glyceryl Stearate (and) PEG-100 Stearate	8.00
C	Aluminum Zirconium Tetrachlorohydrex GLY, 30% Soln.	33.00
	Aluminum Chloride, 32° Baume Soln.	5.50
	Aluminum Chlorhydrate, 50% Soln.	16.50
D	Cyclomethicone	7.00
E	Fragrance, Dye, Preservative	q.s.

Add VEEGUM HV to water at 75° C and mix with maximum available shear until smooth, uniform and completely free of undispersed particles. In another container, heat B to 75° C. Heat C to 55° C in a third container. Add B to A with slow mixing and cool to 50° C. Add C to A & B. Mix at slow speed until the temperature reaches 25° C. Add D and homogenize for 5 minutes. Add E. Mix until uniform and package.

CONSISTENCY: Viscosity measured after 30 days at room temperature is 600-800 cps using Brookfield Model LV, Spindle 3 at 60 rpm. pH: 3.3-3.7.

SUGGESTED PACKAGING: Roll-On Containers

#2

A	VEEGUM	1
	Water	51
B	ARLACEL 165	8
C	Chlorhydrol	20
	Water	20
	Preservative	q.s.

Add the VEEGUM to the water slowly, agitating continually until smooth and heat to 70° C. Heat (B) to 75° C. and add to (A). Mix until 50° C. Dissolve the Chlorhydrol in the Water and heat to 50° C. Add (C) to other components. Mix until cool.

#3

1.	Water (deionized)	50.9
2.	Sequestrene NA2	0.1
3.	Propylene Glycol U.S.P.	3.0
4.	BENTONE™ LT	0.5
5.	ARLACEL 165	7.5
6.	CERASYNT 840	2.5
7.	Methylparaben U.S.P.	0.2
8.	Perfume	0.3
9.	Chlorhydrol (50% sol'n)	35.0

Add items (1), (2), and (3) to a suitable stainless steel steam jacketed kettle and heat to 60°C. Using a homomixer at medium speed (1200 rpm), add item (4), and mix for 20 minutes until well dispersed. Add to this mixture item (5), (6), and (7) and heat to 75°C while stirring slowly. When waxes are completely melted, remove heat and stir at medium speed. Add item (8) at 50°C and mix in. Add item (9) slowly at 45°C and mix in. Continue stirring until lotion reaches room temperature (avoid unnecessary air entrapment).

Antiperspirant Gel

A	BRIJ 56	15.0
	BRIJ 98	10.0
	Mineral Oil	5.0
B	Chlorhydrol 50% W/W Solution	40.0
C	Aluminum Chlorhydroxy Allantoinate	0.3
	Distilled Water	29.2
D	Perfume Oil	0.5

Slowly stir (B) at 80° C into (A) at 80°C. Add (C) heated to 70°C. and at 50° C. add (D).

Antiperspirant Cream

#1

Part A	Mineral Oil	10.0
	IONOL C.P.	0.1
	MONAMID 150-IS	2.0
Part B	Chlorhydrol 50%	40.0
	MONAWET SNO-35	1.4
	Water, deionized	46.5

Mix Part A and Part B separately, in the order listed, then add Part B to Part A with rapid mechanical stirring. This cream is a heavy, water-in-oil emulsion which has excellent stability.

	No.2	No.3
Sodium Aluminum Chlorhydroxy Complex (40% solution)	50.0	50.0
Specially Denatured Alcohol	42.0	42.0
Propylene Glycol	3.0	3.0
Sodium Stearate	6.0	
Sodium Hydroxide		0.75
Stearic Acid		5.25
Water		2.0
Perfume	q.s.	q.s

The aqueous Aluminum Salt Solution is heated to 60-65° C. and the Alcohol and Propylene Glycol slowly added with agitation and added heat to maintain the temperature. The sodium Stearate is added with stirring until the soap dissolves. The Perfume is finally added and, after thorough mixing, the solution is poured into molds.

In the second mixture, with Sodium Stearate formed in situ, the Stearate Acid is dissolved in the warmed Alcohol, the Sodium Hydroxide is dissolved in the Water and the alkali solution is about the same temperature which is added with stirring. the formulation of the soap takes place rapidly and after slight cooling the Perfume is mixed in the solution poured into molds. There is little or no difference in result if the alcoholic solution is added to the aqueous or vice versa, but Stearic Acid must be dissolved in the Alcohol and the alkali in water.

4

(Oil -in-Water)

A	Stearic Acid (triple pressed)	14
	Beeswax	2
	Mineral Oil	1
	ARLACEL 60	5
	TWEEN 60	5
B	Water	33
C	Aluminum Chlorhydroxide (50% aqueous solution)	40
	Perfume	q.s.

Heat (A) to 85° C, (B) to 85° C. Add (B) to (A) while stirring. Mix while cooling to 40° C. Add (C) and continue mixing until cool.

5

(Oil-in-Water)

A	Cetyl Alcohol	5
	ARLACEL 165	5
B	Water	50
	Aluminum Chlorhydroxide (50% aqueous solution)	40

Heat (A) to 70° C, (B) to 72° C. Add (B) to (A) with agitation. Stir until cream has set.

Deodorant Stick

A	VANSEAL CS	30.0
	Sodium Hydroxide (20% sol'n.)	2.0
	Cetyl Alcohol	21.4
	Glycerin	4.0
B	Carbowax 6000	16.8
	Stearic Acid	20.0
	Propylene Glycol	5.3
C	VANCIDE TBS	0.5

Blend (A) over low heat until melted. Add (B) to (A) stirring over low heat until melted. Add (C) stirring until VANCIDE TBS goes into solution. Pour into stick mold while hot and allow to cool.

Chapter II
HAIR PRODUCTS

Shampoo

#1

(High Performance Family)

	% Weight	% Active
Water, preservative	28.3	-
Hexylene Glycol	1.0	-
MONAMATE OPA-30	35.0	9.5
Alpha Olefin Sulfonate (40%)	15.3	6.1
MONATERIC LMM-30	20.4	6.1
	100.0	21.7

Add ingredients in order listed while blending.

Properties:
pH adjusted to 6.6 Viscosity = 1800 cps.

#2
(Basic Family)

	% Weight	% Active
Water and preservative	48.7	-

Alpha Olefin Sulfonate (40%)	25.0	10.0
MONATERIC CDX-38	26.3	10.0
	100.0	20.0

Add ingredients in order listed and blend.

Properties:
pH adjusted to 7.0 Viscosity = 20,000 cps

#3

MACKAM J	12.50
Sodium Lauryl Ether Sulfate 60%	6.60
MACKAMIDE C	2.60
DL Panthenol	0.10
Botanical Extracts Blend	q.s.
Citric Acid (Desired pH level as 1% solution)	q.s.
Methyl Paraben	q.s.
Fragrance, Deionized Water	q.s.
MACKSTAT DM	
Sodium Chloride (if necessary only)	q.s.

Blend together at 40 degrees C. with slow mixing to avoid aeration.

Properties:

pH:	6.0
Solids:	12.0
Viscosity:	5300 cps

#4
(All Purpose)

MACKADET SBC-8	20.0
Sodium Chloride	qs
MACKSTAT DM	qs

Water, Dye, Fragrance qs to	100.0

Add MACKADET SBC-8 to water and blend until clear. Add MACKSTAT DM and adjust viscosity to 2000 - 3000 cps with sodium chloride. Add dye, fragrance, and blend until clear.

#5
(Daily)

POLYOX WSR-20	0.25
Ammonium Lauryl Sulfate (28% active)	28.57
Sodium Laureth Sulfate (28% active)	7.14
Lauramide DEA	2.00
Coco-Betaine (43% active)	6.98
Deionized water	55.06
Perfume and preservative	q.s.

Sprinkle POLYOX WSR-205 into room temperature water with moderate to fast propeller agitation. Mix until dissolved. Slow down mixing rate and heat to 60-65°C. Add surfactants and mix until dissolved. Cool to room temperature.

#6
(Mild)

Sodium Laureth Sulfate (30%)	20.0
MACKAMIDE C	2.0
MACKAM 35	4.0
MACKANATE OM	6.0
Sodium Chloride	2.0
MACKSTAT DM	q.s.
Water, Dye, Fragrance qs to	100.0

Add component to water and heat to 40 degrees C. Blend until clear and adjust pH to 6.5-7.0 with citric acid.

#7
(Super Mild)

1. Ammonium Laureth Sulfate 30%	20.0
2. MACKANATE LO-SPECIAL	20.0

3.	MACKAMIDE PKM	4.0
4.	EGDS	1.0
5.	MACKAM 35HP	7.0
6.	Sodium Chloride	1.0
7.	Deionized Water Q.S. to	100.0
8.	MACKAMIDE LLM	q.s.
9.	MACKSTAT DM	q.s.
10.	Fragrance	q.s.

Into mixing tank place #1,2,3,4,5 and 7 start heating to 170 degrees F. (76 degrees C.) Start mixing keep for 20 minutes at 170 degrees F. (76 degrees C.) then start cooling to 90 degrees F. (30 degrees C.) Adjust pH with diluted Sodium Hydroxide solution up to specifications, then add #6. If needed, increase viscosity with Mackamide LLM.

Properties:
pH 6-7
Misc. 1000-4000cps

#8
(Adult "One Step")

	% Weight	% Active
Water and Preservative	30.0	-
MONAMATE OPA-30	35.0	9.5
MONATERIC 985A	35.0	12.2
	100.0	21.7

Add ingredients in order listed, while blending.

Properties:
pH = 6.5 Viscosity = 1600 cps.

#9
(Mild Salon)

MACKANATE OM	20.0
MACKANATE CP	10.0

Sodium Laureth Sulfate (30%)	20.0
MACKAM 35HP	5.0
Sodium Chloride qs to	5,000cps
MACKSTAT DM	qs
Water, Fragrance, Dye qs to	100.0

Add surfactants to water and heat to 50 degrees C. Blend until clear and add remaining components. Adjust viscosity and cool.

#10
(Extra Mild With Aloe)

Deionized Water	37.50
Aloe Vera Gel	25.00
Lauramide DEA	12.00
VANSEAL CS	5.50
TEA Lauryl Sulfate	20.00
Preservative, color, fragrance	q.s.

Add Aloe Vera Gel to the water with gentle stirring. Add each ingredient in order allowing sufficient stirring time to become clear and uniform. No heat is necessary in the preparation of this formula. Mixing should be accomplished by using a method which minimizes air entrapment.

Properties:
CONSISTENCY: Pourable liquid. (Viscosity - 1300-1600 cps; Brookfield Model LVT, spindle 3 at 60 rpm, measured after 30 days at room temperature.)

SUGGESTED PACKAGING: Squeeze bottle.

#11
(All Natural)

MACKADET WGS	45.0
MACKAMIDE LLM	10.0

Sodium Chloride	2.5
MACKSTAT DM	q.s.
EDTA (40%)	0.5
Fragrance	q.s.
Deionized Water Q.S.	100.0

Add components to water and blend until clear. If a higher viscosity is neede, adjust with sodium chloride.

#12
(Animal Free)

MACKADET 40K	50.0
MACKAMIDE LLM	10.0
Sodium Chloride	2.0
Tetrasodium EDTA (40%)	1.0
MACKSTAT DM	q.s.
Deionized Water q.s. to	100.0

Add MACKADET 40K, MACKAMIDE LLM, and EDTA to 90 percent of the water. Blend until clear. Dissolve Sodium Chloride in remaining water and slowly add to batch. Add MACKSTAT DM and blend until clear. If needed, sodium chloride can be increased to increase viscosity.

#13
(Liquid)

Ammonium Lauryl Sulfate	24.00
MACKAMIDE C	4.95
MACKAM J	8.40
Glycerin	3.00
Deionized Water, Fragrance, Color	q.s.
MACKSTAT DM	q.s.
Citric Acid (1% solution to desired pH level)	q.s.

Blend together at 35-40 degrees C. slowly.
Properties:

pH:	6.4
Solids:	19.0
Viscosity:	7700 cps

#14
(Clear Clean)

Sodium Laureth Sulfate (30%)	25.0
MACKANATE EL	12.0
MACKAMINE CAO	5.0
MACKALENE 426	4.0
MACKSTAT DM	q.s.
Sodium Chloride qs to 2000 cps	
Citric Acid to pH 6.0 - 7.0	
Water, Fragrance qs to	100.0

Blend components and heat to 40 degrees C. Adjust viscosity with sodium chloride and pH with citric acid. Add fragrance and cool.

#15
(Crystal Clear With Silicone Sulfosuccinate)

1.	Sodium Lauryl Sulfate 30%	25.00
2.	MACKAM CB-35	10.00
3.	MACKANATE DC - 30	2.25
4.	MACKSTAT DM	q.s.
5.	D.I. Water	q.s.
6.	Fragrance	q.s.
7.	Disodium EDTA	0.2
8.	Sodium Chloride	q.s.

To the water add #7 start mixing add #1, #2, #3 mix. Add #4, #6 and mix until homogeneous. Adjust viscosity by adding very small portions of #7.
Properties:
pH 6.6 - 6.9 (adjust with diluted hydrochoric acid)

Viscosity 1000 - 3000

#16

(Viscous Clear)

Sodium Lauryl Sulfate (30%)	31.0
MACKAM CAP	6.0
MACKAMIDE C	1.0
MACKPRO NLP	1.0
Disodium EDTA	0.1
Sodium Chloride	1 - 2.0
MACKSTAT DM	q.s.
Deionized Water, Fragrance, Dye qs to	100.0

Add surfactants to water and slow mixing. Use gentle heat until all components are completely and clearly dissolved. Then add MACKPRO NLP and mix. Add MACKSTAT DM, fragrance and dye. Check pH and adjust with Citric Acid. Adjust viscosity with the salt (Sodium Chloride) dissolved in a little water.

Properties:

pH	5.8 - 6.8
Viscosity (cps 25 degrees C.)	8000 - 12000

#17

(Viscous, Low Cost)

	% Weight	% Active
Water and Preservative	78.9	-
NEODOL 25-3A	8.6	5.0
MONAMINE 779	10.0	10.0
MONAMID 150-ADY	2.5	2.5
	100.0	17.5

Add ingredients in order listed and mix with slow agitation. Adjust pH level. At pH 7 viscosity is approximately 5000 cps.

#18

(Economy)

MACKADET SBC-8	10.0
Sodium Chloride	q.s.

MACKSTAT DM	q.s.
Water, Dye, Fragrance qs to	100.0

Add MACKADET SBC-8 to water and blend until clear. Add MACKSTAT DM and adjust viscosity to 3000 - 4000 cps with sodium chloride. Add dye and fragrance and blend until clear.

#19

(Clean Scalp Type)

1.	MACKAM 2C	28.00
2.	Sodium Laureth Sulfate 28%	36.00
3.	MACKAMIDE LLM	4.00
4.	Laneth 15 or Laneth 16	1.00
5.	Propylene Glycol	3.00
6.	Disodium EDTA	0.20
7.	Hydrolyzed Animal Protein 100%	1.00
8.	Methyl Paraben	0.14
9.	Propyl Paraben	0.07
10.	GERMALL 2	0.40
11.	Botanical Extract Blend	q.s.
12.	Color, Fragrance (if required)	q.s.
13.	Deionized Water (qs to)	100.00

PROCEDURE:
Place a major portion of water #13, into manufacturing tank and start heating to 160 degrees F (70 degrees C) Add #6. Start the mixing. Then add #1, #2, #3, #4 slowly. In a separate container heat the remainder of the water #13 to 160 degrees F (70 degrees C) and dissolve in it #8, #9 and add the hot solution to the heated main batch in the tank. Start cooling and at 120 degrees F (50 degrees C) add #7, then #10. Keep mixing and add at 105 degrees F (40 degrees C) #11 and finally #12 (if required). Mix till cool. Check pH and adjust if needed downward with Citric acid or upward with diluted Sodium Hydroxide solution in small increments. Adjust viscosity upwards with very small amounts of salt.

Properties:

pH	7.9 - 8.2
Solids	35%

Viscosity 600-800 CPS at 25 degrees C.

#20

(Moisturizing)

MACKANATE NLD	20.0
Sodium Laureth Sulfate (25%)	18.0
MACKAM NLP	4.0
MACKALENE NLC	1.5
Sodium chloride	q.s.
MACKSTAT DM	q.s.
Water, Fragrance, Dye qs to	100.0
Citric Acid to pH = 5.5 - 6.0	

Add components to water and heat to 40 degrees C. Blend until clear. Adjust viscosity to 3,000 cps with sodium chloride. Cool and fill.

#21

("Beer")

Beer (Flat)	33.3
Sodium Olefin Sulfonate	22.5
Sodium Laureth Sulfate	15.0
MACKAM 35HP	12.0
PEG 150 Distearate	2.0
Ammonium Chloride	1.0
MACKSTAT DM	q.s.
Citric Acid to pH 5.3	
Water, Fragrance, Dye qs to	100.00

Add surfactants to water and heat to 60 degrees C. Blend until clear. Cool to 40 degrees C. and add Beer. Adjust pH and add remaining components.

#22

(Awapuhi Extract Type)

1. Sodium Laureth Sulfate 60%	18.5
2. MACKAMIDE C	4.3
3. Linoleic Acid	1.4-1.7
4. MACKAM J (or MACKAM 35 plus salt)	3.0
5. MACKAM HV	3.0

6.	Hydrolyzed Animal Keratin	1.0
7.	MACKERNIUM 007	1.0
8.	DL Panthenol	0.05-0.1
9.	Citric Acid	q.s.
10.	Lactic Acid	q.s.
11.	Methyl Paraben	q.s.
12.	Propyl Paraben	q.s.
13.	Quaternium 15	q.s.
14.	Plant Extract	q.s.
15.	Fragrance	q.s.

Place warm #14 into the tank and add #11, #12, and dissolve with mixing. To the solution add #1 thru #5 and dissolve with mixing. Add #6, #7, #8 add #9, #10 to obtain correct pH. While mixing add #13 then #15. Blend everything together uniformly with mixing. Adjust viscosity if needed with salt.

Properties:

pH	6.3
Solids, %:	20.0
Viscosity:	10.000 cps

#23

(High Foaming 2 in 1)

Ammonium Lauryl Sulfate (28%)	65.0
MACKALENE 426	6.0
MACKANATE DC-30	4.0
Ethylene Glycol Distearate	1.0
MACKAMIDE PKM	2.0
MACKERNIUM 007	0.4
MACKSTAT DM	q.s.
Water, Dye, Fragrance qs to	100.0

Combine the first five components and heat to 70 degrees C. with continuous mixing. Dilute the MACKERNIUM 007 in the remaining water and slowly add to the blend. Blend until product is homogenous and cool to

50 degrees C. Add MACKSTAT DM, fragrance and dye. Adjust pH with citric acid to 5.0 - 6.0 and cool.

#24

(High Foaming)

Part A

Deionized Water	57.3
Disodium EDTA	0.1
Ammonium Lauryl Sulfate	25.0
CROSULTAINE C-50	10.0

Part B

GERMABEN II	1.0
INCROMIDE CAC	5.0
Perfume (H/47120-Robertet)	0.5
BHT	0.1

Part C

CROQUAT WKP	0.5
KERASOL	0.5

Combine the water and Disodium EDTA of Part A with mixing. When uniform, add the remaining ingredients of Part A. Combine ingredients of Part B with mixing and heat to 45°C if necessary to dissolve the BHT. Add Part B to Part A with mixing. Add ingredients of Part C in order with mixing. Adjust pH if necessary with a 10% citric acid solution.

Properties:
pH to 6.5 w/citric acid - 10%
Viscosity 11,900cps RVT Sp. #5 @ 20rpm, 1 min. 25°C.

#25

(High Foaming 2 in 1 with Selenium Disulfide)

1.	Ammonium Lauryl Sulfate 28%	60.00
2.	MACKALENE 426	9.30
3.	MACKANATE DC30	3.70
4.	Ethylene Glycol Distearate	1.85

5.	MACKAMIDE S	1.50
6.	Selenium Disulfide Powder	1.00
7.	5% solution of Hydroxyethyl Cellulose in water	10.00
8.	5% suspension of Magnesium Aluminum Silicate	10.00
9.	AEROSIL	1.50
10.	Lauryl Alcohol	0.50
11.	Diethanolamine to pH of 5 to 6	q.s.
12.	MACKSTAT DM	q.s.
13.	Fragrance	q.s.
14.	Color solution Blue	q.s.

Into stainless steel mixing tank measure #1, #2, #3, #4. Start heating and slow mixing and heat to 70°C (160°F) In a separate stainless or glass container blend #6 and #5 at room temperature until a smooth uniform paste is formed which will eventually be added later on.

In another container prepare the 5% suspension #8 and mix the suspension till it is completely uniform and viscous and shows no undissolved particles. Preserve suspension if not used immediately with some #12.

In another container prepare the % solution of #7 using heat and mix well until a perfectly sparkling clear viscous solution results. Preserve if not used immediately with a little of #12.

When the temperature in the main mixing tank has reached 70°C (160°F) mix the suspension #8 and solution #7 together and heat to 70°C (160°F) and add to the main tank while continuously mixing well. Be sure that there are no undissolved particles in the #1, #2, #3, #4 before the addition of the suspension #8 and the solution #7. Add #10.

After everything is well blended together add slowly the blend of #6 and #5 to the main tank.

After the blending of all ingredients at the high temperature has proceeded well start sprinkling the very fine flakes of #3 and with very good mixing, to obtain a very smooth creme, start cooling and at 50°C (120°F) add #12 and finally 13. Cool a sample out of the batch and check pH if necessary add #11 to adjust.
As color we tested a solution of DC Blue #2 which seems to be stable.

Properties:
pH 5.2 - 6.4
Viscosity 5000 -10000 CPS

#26
(Cream)

MACKANATE LO-SPECIAL	88.0
MACKOL 16	2.0
BRIJ 52	2.0
MACKSTAT DM	q.s.
Water, Fragrance qs to	100.0

Add MACKOL 16, Brij 52 and water to MACKANATE LO-SPECIAL and heat to 70 degrees C. Blend until homogenous. Adjust pH to 5.5 to 6.0 with sodium hydroxide. Cool to 50 degrees C. and add MACKSTAT DM and fragrance. Adjust solid to 40.0 ± 1.0 at this point. Cool and fill.

Properties:

Solids, %:	40.0
pH (as is):	5.5
Appearence:	Pearly Cream

#27
(Gel)

Sodium Lauryl Ether Sulfate 60%	24.00
MACKAM OB-30	14.50
MACKAMIDE LLM	4.00
Fragrance, Color, Deionized Water	q.s.
Polysorbate 20	q.s.
Propylene Glycol	q.s.
MACKSTAT DM	q.s.
Citric Acid (1% solution to desired pH level)	q.s.

Blend together at 45 degrees C. with slow mixing to avoid aeration.

Properties:

pH:	6.1

Solids:	25.5
Viscosity Approx:	15.000 cps

#28

(Gel)

Part A	
Deionized Water	44.75
TEA Lauryl Sulfate	20.00
INCROSUL OTS	20.00
INCRODET TD-7C	2.00
INCRONAM 30	5.00
INCROMECTANT AQ	3.00
Part B	
INCROMIDE LR	3.00
CROTHIX	1.25
Part C	
GERMABEN II	1.00

Combine ingredients of Part A with mixing and heat to 65°C. Combine ingredients of Part B with mixing and heat to 60°C. Add Part B, to Part A with mixing and cool to 40°C. Add Part C with mixing and cool to desired fill temperature.

Properties:
pH 6.2
Viscosity RV 7 @ 25°C, 20 rpm, 120,000 cps

#29

(Aloe Vera Gel)

Aloe Vera Gel Liquid (1:1)	50.0
Water	14.5
MACKERNIUM 007	3.0
MACKADET SBC-8	32.0
MACKSTAT DM	q.s.
Fragrance, Dye qs to	100.0

Disperse MACKERNIUM 007 in water and Aloe Vera Liquid. Add MACKADET SBC-8 and heat to 45 degrees C. Blend until homogenous.

Adjust viscosity with sodium chloride. Add remaining components and blend until clear. Cool and fill.

#30

(Low pH, Protein Gel)

Ammonium Lauryl Sulfate (30%)	35.0
MACKAM 35HP	12.0
MACKPRO NLP	2.0
MACKAMIDE LLM	2.0
MACKSTAT DM	q.s.
Lactic Acid	q.s.
Water, Dye, Fragrance qs to	100.0

Add first four components to water and heat to 60 degrees C. Adjust pH to 5.0 with lactic acid. Cool and add remaining components at 40 degrees C.

#31

(Pearlescent Luxury)

MONAMATE LNT-40	25.0
Sodium Lauryl Sulfate (28%)	55.0
MONAMID 1089	5.0
CERASYNT IP	0.5
Preservative	0.3
H_3PO_4(85%)	0.4
Water	13.8

Mix Sodium Lauryl Sulfate, water and preservative. Add H_3PO_4. Stir and add MONAMID 1089. Stir until homogeneous and add MONAMATE LNT-40. Add Cerasynt IP. Stir and heat to completely melt the solid material (approx. 60°C). Cool with stirring. At ∠ 40°C add any perfume or colors. Continue stirring and cooling to 25°C. Adjust pH to 6.0-7.0.

Properties:

Appearance	Pearly liquid
Nominal Activity	31 %
Viscosity	4000-5000 cps.

#32

(Highly Pearlescent)

Sodium Lauryl Ether Sulfate 60%	20.0
MACKAMIDE C	2.0
MACKESTER SP	2.0
Stearic Acid	2.0
Magnesium Sulfate (7 $H_2 0$)	6.0
Diethanolamine	0.67
MACKSTAT DM	q.s.
Deionized Water, Fragrance, Dye qs to	100.0

Heat water to 75 degrees C. and add Magnesium Sulfate. Dissolve completely then add other surfactants and DEA then add waxes. Keep temperature at 70 degrees C. for 20 minutes start cooling slowly. At 35 degrees C. add remainder of ingredients and cool while mixing to room temperature. Adjust pH with DEA or Sulfuric Acid diluted solutions.

Properties:
pH 7.5-8.0
Viscosity (cps 25 degrees C)

#33

(Pearly)

1. Ammonium Laureth Sulfate 27%	40.00
2. MACKALENE 426	4.00
3. MACKAMIDE PKM	3.00
4. Ethylene Glycol Di-Stearate	1.50
5. MACKERNIUM 007	0.60
6. MACKSTAT DM	q.s.
7. Color, Fragrance	q.s.
8. Magnesium Sulfate (Epsom Salt)	1.00
9. Sodium Cloride	0.30
10. Deionized Water Q.S. to	100.00

Place #1, #2, #3 and #4 into the stainless steel mixing tank, equipped with a slow speed mixing agitator. Start heating the contents to 170 degrees F. Start slow speed mixing and add D.I. Water 170 degrees hot. In a part of the hot water dissolve #8 and #9 and add to the blend in the batch tank and mix in for 10-15 minutes. Then start fast cooling, mix in #5 at 113 degrees F. and #6 and #7 at 105 degrees F. Let the product stay for a few hours (or over night) without mixing then fill. Addition of more of #9 will thin out solution if it is too viscous.

Properties:

pH	5.5-6.5

#34

(Emulsified Pearly)

1.	MACKADET CA	30.00
2.	Glycerin	1.30
3.	MACKESTER EGMS	1.50
4.	MACKERNIUM 007	2.50
5.	MACKSTAT DM	q.s.
6.	Fragrance, Color	q.s.
7.	Sodium Chloride	1.50
8.	Deionized Water Q.S. to	100.00

Into stainless steel tank put #8 then #1, #2, #3 and heat to 75 degrees C. Start mixing and keep the temperature at 75 degrees C. until everything is completely dissolved. Start cooling and at 50 degrees C. add #4 while mixing; continue mixing while cooling and at 35 degrees C. add #5. Then add #6, leave cool solution standing so that pearlescent can develp and then add #7 (dissolve in a very small amount of water) mix in.

Properties:
pH 6.6-7.4
Viscosity 7000 - 14.000 cps

#35

(Pearly Silver for Gray or White Hair)

MACKADET SBC-8	40.0
MACKAM J	5.0

Glycerine	2.0
MACKESTER SP	1.3
MACKANATE DC-30	1.0
DC Violet #2	q.s.
DC External Violet #2	q.s.
Water, Fragrance	q.s.
MACKSTAT DM	q.s.

Heat water to 180 degrees F. add melted MACKESTER SP and mix. Add MACKADET SBC-8, keep heat at 180 degrees F. until all is dissolved. Mix 15 minutes, start slow cooling. Add glycerine at 150 degrees and then add MACKAM J mix to 110 degrees F. Add MACKANATE DC-30 and then add MACKSTAT DM and fragrance. Dissolve colors in a little of above mixture and add to batch. Cool to room temperature. Check pH, adjust to 6.8 with citric acid. Add salt to thicken.

#36
(Conditioning)

	% Weight	% Active
Water, preservative	62.7	-
POLYMER JR 400	0.8	-
MONATERIC 805	25.0	10.0
MONATERIC ISA-35	10.0	3.5
MONAMID 1034	1.5	1.5
	100.0	15.0

Dissolve Polymer JR400 in water while warming to 50°C. When clear add remaining ingredients. Cool, adjust pH level.

Properties:
pH adjusted to 7.0
Viscosity 500 to 1000 cps.

#37
(Conditioning Shampoo)

Water	45.15
SIPON ES-2	20.00
MONATERGE 1164	20.00

PHOSPHOTERIC QL-38	10.00
DOW CORNING 200 FLUID	2.50
KESSCO ETHYLENE GLYCOL DISTEARATE	1.00
MONAMID CMA	1.00
Sodium Chloride	0.15
GERMABEN II	0.20

Excluding Germaben II, add ingredients in order listed with agitation. Heat to 70°C. Cool to 40°C. Adjust pH to 5.50-6.0 with 50% citric acid. Add Germaben II.

#38
(Conditioning)

MACKANATE LO-SPECIAL	83.0
MACKAMIDE PKM	4.0
MACKPRO NLP	2.0
MACKERNIUM 007	0.8
MACKSTAT DM	q.s.
Water, Fragrance qs to	100.0

Add MACKAMIDE PKM and MACKPRO NLP to MACKANATE LO-SPECIAL and heat to 70 degrees C. Blend until homogenous. Dissolve MACKERNIUM 007 in water and add to product. Blend until completely homogenous. Cool to 50 degrees C. with mild agitation. Add MACKSTAT DM and fragrance and cool with continous agitation.

#39
(Conditioning)

MACKAM 35	35.0
MACKALENE 116	10.0
POLYMER JR30M	1.2
MACKSTAT DM	q.s.
Water, Dye, Fragrance qs	100.0

Disperse Polymer JR30M in cold water. Heat to 60 degrees C. with agitation. Stir until lumps are dissolved. Add MACKAM 35 and MACKALENE 116. Cool to 45 degrees C. and add remaining components.

#40
(Conditioning)

Part A

INCRONAM 30	5.0
INCROMIDE LR	5.0
CRODAFOS SG	3.0
CROVOL PK-70	1.0
SLES (3 mole)	20.0
Deionized Water	64.0

Part B

CROSILKQUAT	1.0
GERMABEN II	1.0

Combine ingredients of Part A with mixing and heat to 75°C. Cool with mixing to 40°C and Part B. Continue mixing and cool to desired fill temperature.

Properties:
pH=4.5
Viscosity Brookfield RV#3 @ 5rpm=8900cps

#41
(Mild Conditioning)

MACKANATE EL	10.0
MACKAM 35	25.0
Sodium Laureth Sulfate (60%)	10.0
MACKANATE DC-30	1.0
MACKAMIDE C	2.0
Polysorbate 20	1.0
MACKSTAT DM	q.s.
Water, Dye, Fragrance qs to	100.0

Add surfactants to water. Start mixing at room temperature until all components are clearly dissolved. Blend fragrance with Polysorbate and add to batch. Adjust pH if necessary with citric acid. Adjust viscosity with Sodium Chlorate.
Properties:
pH 5.5-6.7
Viscosity (cps 25 degrees C.) 600 - 1200

#42
(Non-Irritating and
Mildly Conditioning)

MONATERIC 985A	40.00
MONAMATE OPA-30	30.00
CERASYNT IP	2.00
Preservative*	0.30
H_3PO_4(85%)	0.75
Water	26.95

Mix MONATERIC 985A, MONAMATE OPA-30, water, Preservative and Cerasynt IP. Heat with stirring to completely melt the solid materials (approx. 60°C). Add H_3PO_4. Cool with stirring. At ∠ 40°C add any perfume or colors. Continue stirring and cooling to 25°C. Adjust pH to 6.5 - 7.0.

Properties:

Appearence	Pearly viscous liquid
Nominal Activity	26%

#43
(Supermild Conditioning)

MACKANATE CP SPECIAL	25.0
Sodium laureth-1 Sulfate (30%)	25.0
MACKESTER EGMS	1.0
MACKLALENE 426	4.0
MACKAMIDE LLM	3.0
MACKAM 35HP	4.0
Sodium Chloride	q.s. to 2 - 5 m cps

MACKSTAT DM	0.4
Water	q.s. to 100.0

Add components (except NaCl and DM) to water and heat to 70°C. Blend until homogenous. Cool to 50°C and add NaCL and Mackstat DM. Adjust pH to 6.0 - 6.5 with citric acid and add fragrance.

#44

(Daily Conditioning)

Water	42.1
MONATERIC L-30	40.0
MONATERIC LMAB	13.3
MONATERIC 1203	3.3
MONAMID 1007	1.3

Add ingredients as listed (no heat required). Mix until uniform. Adjust pH to 6.5-7.5. Add preservative as required.

Properties:

Appearence	Clear viscous liquid
Nominal Activity	18.5%

#45

(Daily Conditioning for Oily Hair)

UCARE POLYMER JR-400	0.5
SOLULAN 16	2.0
SOLULAN 98	1.0
Ammonium Lauryl Sulfate (28%)	60.0
Cocamidopropylamine Oxide (30%)	5.0
Citric Acid (40% Aq. Solution)	q.s. to pH 5-6
Deionized water	31.5
Perfume and preservative	q.s.

Disperse Ucare Polymer JR-400 in water at room temperature. When well dispersed, heat to 65°C. When clear, add ammonium lauryl sulfate, cocamidopropylamine oxide and SOLULAN 98, in this order, mixing until clear and uniform after addition of each material. Separately, heat SOLULAN 16 to 50°C. Add SOLULAN 16 at 50°C to rest of formula, mix with stirring until clear. Cool to room temperature and adjust pH with citric acid solution to pH 5-6.

#46

(Acid Balanced Conditioning)

TEA Lauryl sulfate (40%)	35.0
MACKAM 35HP	10.0
MACKALENE 426	6.0
MACKSTAT DM	q.s.
Water, Dye, Fragrance qs to	100.0

Add components to water and heat to 40 degrees C. Blend until clear. Adjust pH to 4.0 with citric acid. Cool and fill.

#47

(Clear Conditioning)

	% Weight	% Active
Water, preservative	40.9	-
MONATERIC LMAB	33.3	10.0
MONATERIC ISA-35	14.3	5.0
MONAMID 1007	1.5	1.5
MONAQUAT TG	10.0	3.0
	100.0	19.5

Add ingredients in the order listed and blend.

Properties:
pH adjusted to 7.0
Viscosity approximately 2 to 3000 cps.

#48
(Clear Conditioning)

GLUCQUAT 100	1.0
GLUCAMATE DOE-120	3.5
TEA-Lauryl Sulfate (40% active)	25.0
Lauramide DEA	5.0
Deionized water	65.0
Citric Acid	0.5
Perfume and preservative	q.s.

Heat deionized water to 60°C with propeller agitation. Add TEA-lauryl sulfate, lauramide DEA, preservative, GLUCAMATE DOE-120 and citric acid to batch, in that order, waiting for each ingredient to dissolve before adding the next. When clear add GLUCQUAT 100. Cool to room temperature.

#49
(Family Type With Conditioning)

	% Weight	% Active
Water and preservative	55.5	-
MONATERIC LMAB	25.0	7.5
MONATERIC CDX-38	10.1	3.8
Alpha Olefin Sulfonate (40%)	9.4	3.7
	100.0	15.0

Add ingredients in order listed. When blended adjust pH to level desired.
Properties:

pH ajusted to	7.0
Viscosity =	20,000 cps

Rubine Dye Test (3.5) indicates good substantivity.

#50
(Conditioning and Easy Combing Action)

Sodium Lauryl Ether sulfate (60%)	18.0
MACKAMIDE C	3.0
MACKAMIDE S	2.0
MACKAM 35	5.0

Glycerin	2.0
Disodium EDTA	0.1
Polysorbate 20	1.0
MACKANATE DC-30	1.0
Polyquaternium 10 (2% solution)	20.0
MACKSTAT DM	q.s.
Deionized Water, Fragrance, Dye qs to	100.0

Heat water to 50 degrees C. Start adding the surfactants, Disodium EDTA, Glycerin then the Polyquaternium solution, mix until everything is homogeneous and clear. Then add Mackanate DC-30 and finally dissolve fragrance in Polysorbate 20. At 30 degrees C. add MACKSTAT DM, mix to room temperature. Adjust pH if necessary with Citric Acid. Adjust viscosity with Sodium Chloride.

Properties:

pH	5.5-6.5
Viscosity (cps 25 degrees C.)	1000-3000

#51

(Low Foam Conditioning Shampoo)

MACKAM 35	10.0
MACKALENE 117	15.0
MACKPRO NLP	4.0
NATROSOL 250 HHR	0.7
MACKSTAT DM	q.s.
Water, Dye, Fragrance qs to	100.0

Thoroughly disperse the Natrosol in water and heat to 45 degrees C. Add MACKAM 35, MACKALENE 117, and MACKPRO NLP. Blend until clear. Add MACKSTAT DM, fragrance and dye. Cool and fill.

Properties:

Appearance:	Yellow Clear
pH:	5.9
Viscosity:	470 cps

#52

(Natural Conditioning)

Water	41.6
Sodium Chloride	0.4
Sodium Lauryl Sulfate (28%)	35.7
Phosphoric Acid (85%)	0.1
MONAMATE LNT-40	12.5
MONATERIC CAB	6.7
AVAMID 150	3.0

Add ingredients in the order listed with good agitation. Adjust pH to 6.0-7.0. Add preservative, color and perfume as required.

Properties:

Physical Appearance	Crystal clear liquid
Activity	20%
Viscosity	2800 cps

#53

(Conditioning Neutralizing)

Part A

Deionized Water	60.6
TEALS	25.0
Disodium EDTA	0.3

Part B

INCROMIDE LR	3.0
INCROMIDE CAC	1.1
INCROMINE OXIDE BA	2.0
INCRODET TD-7C	6.0

Part C

HYDROTRITICUM 2000	0.5
CRODACEL QS	0.5
GERMABEN II	1.0

Combine ingredients of Part A with mixing and heat to 65-70°C. Add Part B ingredients individually with good mixing and cool to 45°C. Add Part C with mixing and cool to desired fill temperature.

Properties:

pH= 5.25

Viscosity RVT #5 @ 50rpm=680cps

#54
(Self Adjusting Conditioning)

Water	38.5
NaCl	1.0
MONATERIC 1202	7.5
MONAMID 1089	3.0
TEA-Lauryl Sulfate (40%)	50.0

Add ingredients in order listed. Adjust pH to 6.0-7.0 with citric acid. Add preservative as required.

This formulation blends the efficient cleaning of a high concentration of anionic tempered by the conditioning effects of MONATERIC 1202. The result is clean, shiny hair without the build-up or greasy feel usually associated with traditional conditioning agents, and will selectively be more substantive at those sites on the hair where chemical or physical damage has occurred.

Properties:

Appearance	Clear liquid
Nominal Activity	25.6%

#55
(Ultra Pearlescent Conditioning)

A	VEEGUM® Ultra	2.00
	Deionized Water	61.25
B	TIMIRON MP-1001	0.50
C	Sodium Laureth Sulfate	25.00
	MONAMID 716	7.50
	VANSEAL CS	3.75
	Preservative Fragrance	q.s.

Sift VEEGUM Ultra into the water while mixing at 700rpm with a propeller stirrer. Adjust the propeller speed to 1500-1700rpm and mix for 30 minutes. Add the B ingredients and mix for 5 minutes. Adjust the speed to 200 to 500 rpm and add the C ingredients in the order shown, mixing after each addition until smooth and uniform.

Properties:

Viscosity	7000-9000 cps
pH	5.0 ± 0.2
Color	Pearlescent, white

#56

(Wheat Germ Conditioning)

MACKANATE OP	20.0
Sodium Laureth Sulfate (30%)	24.0
MACKANATE WGD	8.0
MACKAM WGB	5.0
Citric Acid to pH = 5.5	
Sodium chloride qs to viscosity = 20000cps	
MACKSTAT DM	q.s.
Water, Dye, Fragrance qs to	100.0

Add surfactants to water and heat to 40 degrees C. Adjust pH to 5.5. Add remaining components and adjust viscosity with sodium chloride.

#57

(With Protein for Damaged Hair)

Phase A	
Water	49.30
Sorbitol	1.00
Glycol Stearate	1.00
Phase B	
Cocamidopropylhdroxysultaine	20.00
Disodium Cocamido MIPA Sulfosuccinate	20.00
Sodium Lauroyl Sarcosinate	5.00
Phase C	
Propyltrimonium Hydrolyzed Collagen (Protetein)	2.00
Phase D	
GERMABEN II	1.00
Citric Acid	0.50

Fragrance	0.10
FD&C Yellow #5 (0.01% Solution)	0.10

Heat water to 80°C, add Phase A in order listed. Mix until clear. Add Phase B ingredients in order and mix until homogenous. Cool to room temperature. Add Protectein slowly, mix until smooth. Add Phase D ingredients and mix until uniform.

#58

(Damaged Hair)

UCARE Polymer LR-400	0.40
UCARE Polymer LR-30M	0.40
Glucamate SSE-20	3.00
Triethanolamine Lauryl Sulfate (40%)	17.50
Sodium Laureth Sulfate (28%)	17.86
Disodium Laurethsulfosuccinate (40%)	7.50
Lauramide DEA	2.00
Tetrasodium EDTA	0.10
Deionized water	51.24
Perfume and preservative	q.s.

Add Ucare Polymers to water at room temperature with good agitation. Once hydrated add the disodium Laureth-sulfosuccinate. Begin heating and add TEALS and SLES. When at 60-65°C, add the melted GLUCAMATE SSE-20 and lauramide DEA. Upon complete solution, cool to room temperature and add the tetrasodium EDTA.

#59

(Snarl-Free Conditioner)

	% Weight	% Active
Water, preservative	50.8	-
POLYMER JR 400	1.0	1.0
MONATERIC CEM-38	42.2	16.0
MONAMID 716	5.0	5.0
CERAPHYL 60	1.0	0.4

	100.0	22.4

Blend Polymer JR400 into water while heating to 50°C and stir until dispersed and clear. Then add remaining ingredients.

Properties:
at pH 7 viscosity is approximately 500 cps.

#60

(Detangling)

1.	Sodium Lauryl Ether Sulfate 60%	25.00
2.	MACKAM J	5.00
3.	MACKAMIDE S	3.00
4.	Glycerin	2.00
5.	Hydrolyzed Animal Protein 55%	1.00
6.	MACKERNIUM 007	3.50
7.	Polysorbate 20	1.00
8.	Tetrasodium EDTA (40% solution)	0.10
9.	MACKSTAT DM	q.s.
10.	Hydrochloric Acid (1 part acid plus 4 parts of water)	0.5-1.0
11.	Fragrance	q.s
12.	Color	q.s.
13.	Sodium Chloride to adjust viscosity	0.1-0.5
14.	Deionized water	100.00

Into the stainless steel manufacturing tank meter #14 start heating. Add #8 then #1, #2, #3, #4 with mixing and mix until everything is completely dissolved and the solution clear at 120 F. stop heating and add #5 and #6. Separately blend #7 and #11 together well. Start cooling while mixing and at about 90 F. add fragrance blend #7 and #11 then check and adjust pH. By adding the diluted hydrochloric acid solution (slowly add the concentrated acid 1 part to 4 parts of deionized water protecting your eyes and face) in small amount until correct pH is obtained (6.5-7.00) after mixing in. Add #9 and finally small quantities of salt dissolved in a little water until upon mixing the desired viscosity is obtained. Addition of too much salt will thin out the product.

Properties:
pH 6.5 - 7.00

Viscosity 500 - 1500 cps vb

#61

(Detangling, Salt-Free)

MACKAM CAP	20.0
Sodium Laureth Sulfate (60%)	10.0
MACKAMIDE LLM	3.5
Polymer JR	1.4
Disodium EDTA	0.1
MACKSTAT DM	q.s.
Deionized Water, Fragrance, Dye qs to	100.0

Hydrate Polymer JR in water and blend until clear. Slowly add MACKAM CAP and blend until clear. Add Disodium EDTA. Add the remaining components and heat to 45 degrees C. Adjust pH with citric acid if needed.

Properties:

pH	5.5 - 6.5
Viscosity (cps, 25 deg. C.)	10,000 - 20,000

#62

(Super Detangling, Clear)

Sodium Laureth Sulfate (60%)	10.0
MACKAM CAP	20.0
MACKAMIDE LLM	3.5
Tetra Sodium EDTA	0.1
POLYMER JR	1.5
MACKSTAT DM	q.s.
Deionized Water, Fragrance qs to	100

Disperse Polymer JR in water and blend until clear. Add MACKAM CAP, Sodium Laureth Sulfate, MACKAMIDE LLM and Tetra Sodium EDTA. Heat to 40 degrees C. and add remaining components. Blend until clear and adjust pH if necessary. Cool and fill.

#63

(Detangling and Conditioning)

Sodium Lauryl Sulfate	30.0
MACKAMIDE C	2.0
MACKAM CAP	6.0
MACKANATE DC-30	1.0
2% Solution of Polyquaterium 10	60.0
in deionized waterMACKSTAT DM	q.s.
Deionized Water, Fragrance, Dye qs to	100.0

Heat water to 60 degrees C. and add surfactants and start mixing, until solution is uniform and completely clear. Add Polyquaternium 10 solution and blend in then add MACKANATE DC-30. Start cooling while mixing and add remaining components at 30 degrees C. and mix, and cool to room temperature. Adjust pH with Citric Acid and adjust viscosity with Sodium Chloride 1% - 1.5%.

Properties:

pH	5 - 6
Viscosity (cps 25 degrees C.)	600 - 2000

#64

(Amphoteric With Sunscreen)

Phase A

MONAMID 716	1.00
ESCALOL 537Q	0.20

Phase B

Water	47.80
Monateric LMAB	15.00
Maprofix ES-1	35.00

Phase C

GERMABEN II	1.00

Combine Phase A and heat to 80°C, mixing until Escalol 537Q is completely dissolved. Combine Phase B and heat to 80°C. Add Phase A to Phase B.Cool to 50°C and add Phase C. Cool to room temperature.

#65

(Anti-Dandruff)

Water	41.0
TEA-Lauryl Sulfate (40%)	30.0
MONATERIC CAB	17.0
MONAMID 716	3.0
MONAMID 150-ADY	3.0
Zinc Pyrithione (48% Aqueous Dispersion)	4.0
Glycol Distearate	2.0

Add ingredients in order listed. Mix and heat to 60°C. Cool, adjust pH to 6.0. Add coloring, fragrance and preservative as required.

Properties:

Appearance:	Off white, opaque
liquid	
Viscosity:	Approx. 2000 cps.

#66

(Anti-Dandruff)

	% Weight	% Active
Water	22.7	-
MONATERIC CAB	33.3	10.0
MONAMATE OPA-30	37.0	10.0
MONAMID 716	3.0	3.0
MONAMID S	3.0	3.0
Zinc Omadine, 48% Dispersion	1.0	0.5
	100.0	26.5

Procedure: Add first 5 ingredient in the order listed and heat to 97°C with good agitation. Cool to 50°C and blend in the Zinc Omadine.

Properties:

pH =	7.0
Viscosity approx.	10,000 cps

#67

(Anti-Dandruff)

Sodium Olefin Sulfonate	20.0
MACKAM 2C75	16.0
ZINC OMADINE	2.6
MACKOL 16	2.0
MACKAMIDE LLM	2.5
BENTONE EW	0.8
MACKSTAT DM	q.s.
Water, Dye, Fragrance qs to	100.0

Heat water to 70 degrees C. Disperse and homogenize the Bentone EW. Add Zinc Omadine and Mackol 16. Cool to 50 degrees C. and add MACKAM 2C75, AOS and Zinc Omadine. Cool to 40 degrees C. and add remaining components.

#68

(Anti-Dandruff)

MACKAM 2C75	13.0
Sodium Laureth Sulfate	45.0
TEA Lauryl Sulfate (30%)	35.0
MACKAMIDE LLM	2.5
IRGASAN DP 300	0.2
MACKSTAT DM	q.s.
Water, Fragrance, Dye qs to	100.0

Add first four components to water and heat to 50 degrees C. Blend until clear. Add Irgasan DP300. Cool to 40 degrees C. and add remaining components. Cool and fill.

#69

(Anti-Dandruff Cream type)

Sodium Lauryl Sulfate (30%)	61.8
MACKAM 35HP	10.0
Sodium Chloride	7.0
Triple Pressed Stearic Acid	5.0
MACKAMIDE LLM	4.0
Propylene Glycol	4.0
Zinc Pyrithione (48%)	4.0
MACKAMIDE PK	2.0

Caustic Soda (50%)	1.6
MACKSTAT DM	q.s.
Water, Dye, Fragrance qs to	100.0

Heat stearic acid, MACKAMIDE LLM, MACKAMIDE PKM and propylene glycol to 70 degrees C. Heat SLS, MACKAM 35HP, Sodium Chloride, Caustic Soda and water to 70 degrees C. Add oil to water and cool to 55 degrees C. Slowly add Zinc Pyrithione. Cool to 45 degrees C. and add remaining components. Fill at 40 degrees C.

#70

(Anti-Dandruff Lotion)

Part A

VEEGUM	1.0
METHOCEL FYM	0.8
Water qs to	100.0

Part B

Sodium Olefin sulfonate (40%)	35.0
MACKAMIDE LLM	4.0
MACKAMIDE S	1.0
MACKPRO NLP	2.0

Part C

ZINC OMADINE (48%)	4.0

Thoroughly desperse Veegum in water at 70 degrees C. Then slowly add Methocel FYM and blend until homogenous. Add Part B to Part A and adjust pH to 6.5 with citric acid. Add Zinc Omadine and blend until homogenous.

#71

(Antidandruff Sulfur)

A	VEEGUM	1.0
	Water	53.3
B	Colloidal sulfur	1.0
C	SIPON L-22	40.0
	MONAMID 716	4.5
	NaCl	0.2

Preservative	q.s.

Add the VEEGUM to the water slowly, agitating with maximum available shear until smooth. Add B and C in order, mixing after each addition until smooth and uniform. This suspension is prepared without heat in the same manner as the currently popular solution shampoos.

Consistency/Suggested Packaging:
pourable lotion/plastic bottle

#72

(2 In 1 Antidandruff)

1.	Ammonium Lauryl Sulfate	64.00
2.	MACKALENE 426	10.00
3.	MACKANATE DC30	4.00
4.	Ethylene Glycol Distearate	2.00
5.	MACKAMIDE C	1.00
6.	Zinc Pyrithione 50% Suspension	2.00
7.	2% water solution of Hydroxyethyl Cellulose	9.00
8.	5% Dispersion of Magnesium Aluminum Silicate	9.00
9.	MACKERNIUM 007	0.50
10.	MACKSTAT DM	q.s.
11.	Fragrance	q.s.
12.	Color	q.s.
13.	Deionized Water qs to	100.00

Into a stainless steel tank place #1, #2, #3, #4 and start heating and slow mixing and heat to 80°C (176°F). In a separate small stainless vessel, blend #6, and #5 and mix until a smooth uniform paste is formed. Do not add. In a separate container prepare the 2% solution of #7 and mix till solution is completely clear. In another container prepare a 5% suspension of #8 and blend well until the material has formed a completely smooth dispersion free of any particles. Finally blend both, suspension #8 and solution #7, together and then add this blend to the hot batch with good mixing and continue agitation and keep temperature at 70°C (160°F). Once this addition is completed, start addition of blend of #6 in #5 slowly. Keep mixing for 10 minutes then start slow cooling while mixing at 50°C (120°F) then adding #10. Cool further to 35°C (95°F) while mixing and add #11, #12 and enough of #13 to compensate for evaporation. Check pH and adjust with small amounts of diluted sodium hydroxide solution.

DO NOT ADD SALT TO THIS PREPARATION TO INCREASE VISCOSITY .Try only small amounts of additional #5. Adding one half % of Lauryl Alcohol will help. As color you could use very small amounts of FDC Blue #1 solution or FDC Green #3. To prepare #8, we use Magnabrite HV made by American Colloid C. Illinois.

Properties:

pH	5.5 - 6.0
Viscosity	4000 - 5000 cps

#73

(Coal Tar)

1.	Coal Tar Extract *	0.5-5.0
2.	MACKAMIDE ODM	0.25-2.5
3.	MACKADET CA	30.00
4.	MACKSTAT DM	q.s.
5.	Fragrance	q.s.
6.	Deionized Water q.s. to	100.00

Select the desired amount of Coal Tar Extract to be employed in the product.* Register, Part IV, Department of Health and Human Services, 21 CRF Parts 348 and 358.

For each quantity of #1, exactly 1/2 of the #2 material is required to solubilize #1. At cooler temperatures a little warming will be necessary to obtain complete solution. (40 C. 104 F). Into main tank meter add #6 and then #3, Fragrance #5 and finally #4 and mix until everything is completely and uniformly dissolved. Check pH value and adjust with either very small amount of dilute acid downward or a little dilute Sodium Hydroxide upwards.

Properties:

pH	6.6 - 7.4
Viscosity	1000-2000 cps

#74

(Coal Tar and Salicylic Acid)

1.	Coal Tar Extract *	2.5-5.0
2.	Salicylic Acid	1.8-3.0
3.	MACKAMIDE ODM	0.25-2.5

4.	MACKADET CA	50,000
5.	D.I. Water qs to	100.0
6.	20% Sodium Hydroxide Solution qs to	pH 6.5
7.	MACKSTAT DM	q.s.
8.	Fragrance	q.s.

Select to desired amount of #1 to be employed in the product of #2. For each addition of #1 exactly 1/2 of the material #3 is required to solubilize #1 at cooler temperatures or little warming maybe necessary (keep fumes from open flame). Into the main tank meter #5 then add #4 and mix until all is completely dissolved. Add carefully #2 into warm tank (protect eyes, hands) keep mixing until everything is clearly dissolved. Check pH and or adjust upwards by adding small amounts of #6 solution. Add #8 mix to cover odor of #1.

Properties:

pH	6.5-7.3
Viscosity	1000-5000cps

* Federal Register, Part IV, Department of Health and Human Services, 21 CFR Parts 348 and 358.

#75
(Salicylic Acid)

MACKADET CBS	50.0
Salicylic Acid	2.0
MACKSTAT DM	q.s.
Water, Fragrance, Dye qs to	100.0

Disperse Salicylic Acid in the Mackadet CBS and blend until homogenous. Add water and heat to 40 degrees C. Slowly adjust pH to 5.0 with sodium hydroxide and blend until clear. Add remaining components and cool.

#76
(Zinc Pyrithione Lotion)

A	VEEGUM	0.5
	Water	51.1

	JAGUAR HP-60	0.5
B	SIPON L-22	40.0
C	CRODAFOS SG	1.8
	MONAMID 716	4.0
	ZINC OMADINE, 48%	2.1
	Preservative	q.s.

Add the VEEGUM to the water slowly, agitating at maximum available shear until smooth. Add the Jaguar HP-60 and mix until uniformly dispersed. With slow stirring add B. Add the Crodafos slowly and mix until the Jaguar HP-60 is dissolved and smooth. Add the remaining C ingredients in order with slow agitation, mixing until smooth and uniform. Avoid incorporation of air.

Consistency/Suggested Packaging:
pourable lotion/opaque plastic bottle

#77
(Zinc Pyrithione)

A	VEEGUM	1.0
	Water	45.8
	METHOCEL F4M	0.8
B	ZINC OMADINE, 48%	4.2
C	MONAMIDE CMA	5.0
D	MAPROFIX TLS-500	40.0
	Triethanolamine	3.2
	Preservative	q.s.

Heat the water to 70°C. Add VEEGUM to the water slowly, agitating at maximum available shear until smooth. Add the Methocel and continue rapid stirring for an additional 15 minutes. Add B to A and stir rapidly for 5 minutes. Melt C and add with slow stirring. Mix until smooth. Turn off heat and while cooling add D. Mix at slow speed until smooth and uniform.

#78

(Wheat)

Part A	
Deionized Water	48.0
TEALS	30.0
INCROMINE OXIDE WG	5.0
INCRONAM WG-30	5.0
Part B	
INCROMIDE CAC	10.0
Part C	
HYDROTRITICUM 2000	1.0
GERMABEN II	1.0

Combine ingredients of Part A with mixing and heat to 60°C. When clear, add Part B with mixing and cool to 40°C. Add Part C with mixing and cool to desired fill temperature. Adjust pH with a 10% citric acid solution.

Properties:	
Citric Acid to pH	6.5
Brookfield Viscosity, RV#3	50rpm=1580cps

#79

(Medicated Cream)

I.	Stearic Acid (Triple Pressed)	3.5
	NaOH (Flakes)	0.7
	MONAMID 718	6.0
	Water	22.6
	MONATERIC CA-35	10.0
	Sodium Lauryl Sulfate (30%)	50.0
II.	Allantoin	0.2
III.	MONAMID	1.0
	PCMX 716	1.0
IV.	Coal Tar Extract	5.0
	Perfume	q.s.

Blend all ingredients in Part I @ 65-70°C until a homogeneous product is obtained. Add Parts II and III to I. Cool down to 30°C, add Part IV with mixing. A flowable slurry sets up to a paste. Adjust pH to 7.0-8.0.

#80

(Non-Alkaline, 25% Active)

	% As is	% Active
Ammonium Lauryl Sulfate	60.7	17.0
MONAMATE CPA-40%	15.0	6.0
MONATERIC ISA-35%	5.7	2.0
Water (deionized)	18.6	0.0
	100.0	25.0

Weigh out ammonium lauryl sulfate and heat to 50-55°C with slow agitation. Add MONAMATE CPA-40%. Add molten MONATERIC ISA-35% (pumpable at 45-50°C). Add water and allow batch to cool to 40-50°C depending on viscosity. Add perfume, preservative (e.g. methyl paraben) and color as desired. Depending on viscosity, bottle between 25°C and 45°C.

Properties:

pH (as is):	5.8-6.0
Viscosity (CPS) @ 25°C:	4100-4300

#81

(Non-Alkaline)

Ammonium Lauryl Sulfate	25.0
MACKAMIDE LLM	2.0
MACKAM 35	4.0
MACKAM TM	3.0
MACKSTAT DM	q.s
Water, Dye, Fragrance qs to	100.0

Add first four components to water and heat to 50 degrees C. Blend until clear and add hydrochloric acid to pH=5.0. Cool to 40 degrees C. and add remaining components.

#82

(For Permed Hair)

MACKANATE OP	20.0
MACKANATE CP	12.0
Sodium Laureth Sulfate (30%)	15.0
MACKAMINE WGO	4.0
MACKALENE 716	1.0
MACKSTAT DM	q.s.
Citric Acid to pH=6.0	
Sodium chloride qs to 2000cps	
Water, Dye, Fragrance qs to	100.0

Add surfactants to water and heat to 40 degrees C. Blend until clear and adjust pH with citric acid. Add remaining components and adjust viscosity with sodium chloride.

#83

(Neutralizer)

MACKANATE OM	30.0
SODIUM LAURETH SULFATE (30%)	20.0
MACKAMINE CAO	6.0
MACKAMINE WGO	2.0
MACKSTAT DM	q.s.
Water, Dye, Fragrance qs to	100.0

Add surfactants to water and blend until clear. Adjust pH to 5.0-5.5 with citric acid. Add dye and fragrance.

Properties:

Solids, %	19.5
pH	5.3
Viscosity (cps, 25 deg. C.)	1500

#84

(Neutralizing)

MACKADET BSC	30.0
Glycerin 99%	2.0
MACKAM J	2.0
MACKSTAT DM (preservative)	q.s

Fragrance & Color	q.s
Deionized Water qs to	100.0

Blend all ingredients at room temperature. Adjust pH from 4.8-5.5, adjust with sulfate acid if needed.

#85

(Concentrated Conditioning Creme)

1.	MACKADET CA	60.0
2.	Stearic Acid Triple Pressed	7.5
3.	MACKERNIUM 007	7.0
4.	Sodium Hydroxide 20% Solution	5.0-5.5
5.	MACKSTAT DM	q.s
6.	Deionized Water	q.s
7.	Fragrance	q.s

Add #1 into stainless steel creme kettle and start mixing. In separate container separately add #4 to 2/3 of #6 and mix together carefully avoid splashing - PROTECT EYES. Add this solution to creme kettle and start heating to 180 degrees F. (82 degrees C.) with mixing, keep tank well covered. After mixing for 20 min. start cooling, continuing mixing, and at 130 degrees F. (55 degrees C.) add #3 and remainder of #6, keep slowly mixing and cooling. Take sample of warm mixture from tank and take pH reading of cooled sample. Adjust batch if necessary by adding small quantities of solution of #4 to tank if pH is too low or a little diluted citric acid solution if pH is too high. Finally add #5 to tank and then #7 mix for 15 min. and recheck pH and fill at 86 degrees F. (30 degrees C.) into jars.

Properties:

pH	7.2-7.8

#86

(Pearlescent Concentrate)

TEA Lauryl Sulfate	50.0
MACKAMIDE LLM	30.0
MACKESTER SP	5.0

Propylene Glycol	5.0
Sodium Chloride	1.0
Phosphoric Acid to pH = 7.5	
MACKSTAT DM	q.s.
Water, Fragrance, Dye qs to	100.0

Add first five components to water and heat to 70 degrees C. Blend until homogenous. Cool to 40 degrees C. and add MACKSTAT DM, dye and fragrance.

This product can be diluted one pint to a gallon with water. The viscosity can be controlled by regulating the propylene glycol.

#87

(Dilutable Concentrate)

(One Pint to a Gallon)

MACKAMIDE LMD	34.0
Sodium Laureth Sulfate (60%)	29.0
Sodium Olefin Sulfate (40%)	14.0
Propylene Clycol	10.0
Ammonium Chloride	1.5
Citric Acid qs to pH = 6.5	
MACKSTAT DM	q.s.
Water, Dye, Fragrance qs to	100.0

Blend components to water and heat to 50 degrees C. Adjust pH to 6.5. Cool to room temperature.

#88

(Highly Concentrated Detangling)

1.	MACKADET CA	81.50
2.	Tetrasodium EDTA (40% Solution)	0.20
3.	Glycerin	4.00
4.	Hydrolyzed Animal Protein 55% Liquid	2.00
5.	MACKERNIUM 007	7.00
6.	Polysorbate 20	2.00
7.	Fragrance	q.s.
8.	MACKSTAT DM	q.s.

9. Diluted Hydrochloric Acid Solution 1:4	q.s. to pH spec.
10. Color	q.s.
11. Sodium Chloride to adjust viscosity	q.s.
12. Deionized Water q.s. to	100.00

In a stainless steel mixing kettle blend #1, #2, #3 with mixing then add #4 and #5. Slowly mix until all is dissolved, if necessary use a little heating. Adjust pH with the diluted Hydrochloric Acid solution (made by adding 1 part of acid carefully to 4 parts of water (Protecting the Eyes and Face) until correct pH is obtained (6.5-7.0). Add color, if required, add #8 slowly and mix in. If the product is to be sold as concentrate then the quantity of #8 must be increased, fragrance and color also properly increased. If the product is sold diluted then 1 part of the above formula is mixed with 2 parts of deionized water the increased fragrance added then the preservative #8 added at the corrected amount the pH adjusted and finally the salt addition done to obtain the desired viscosity.

Properties:
pH 6.5 - 7.0
Viscosity larger than 1000 cps

#89

(Baby & Family shampoo, 25.8% Active)

Water	12.0
MONAMATE OPA-30	46.3
MONATERIC CSH-32	41.7

Add ingredients in the order listed and blend with slow agitation. No heat is required. Adjust pH with phosphoric acid to 6.0 Viscosity = approximately 600 cps.

#90

(Baby)

1. SIPON ESY	16.00
2. MACKANATE OM	8.00
3. MACKAM 2C	6.00
4. MACKAM J	3.00
5. PARAGON	0.60

6.	Deionized Water	q.s. to 100.00
7.	Color, Fragrance	q.s.

Add components to water and heat to 35°C. Blend until clear. Adjust pH to 6.0-7.0 with citric acid. Adjust viscosity to 1500-5000 cps with NaC1.

#91

(Baby)

Sodium Laureth Sulfate (30%)	15.0
MACKAMIDE C	0.5
MACKAM 35	3.0
MACKANATE OM	5.0
MACKAM 2C	5.0
Sodium Chloride	2.0
MACKSTAT DM	q.s
Water, Dye, Fragrance qs to	100.0

Add components to water and heat to 40 degrees C. Blend until clear. Adjust pH to 6.5-7.0 with citric acid. If needed, adjust viscosity with NaC1.

#92

(Baby)

MACKANATE OM	30.0
Sodium Laureth Sulfate (25%)	17.0
MACKAM 35HP	4.0
Sodium Chloride	3.0
MACKSTAT DM	q.s.
Water, Dye, Perfume qs to	100.0

Add surfactants to water and blend until clear. Adjust pH to 6.5-7.0 with sodium hydroxide or citric acid. Adjust viscosity with sodium chloride. Add dye, preservative and perfume and blend until clear.

Properties:

Solids, %:	17.7
pH:	6.7
Viscosity (cps, 25 degrees C):	1000
Cloud Point:	<5 degrees C.

#93
(Baby)

MACKADET BSC	20.0
MACKSTAT DM	q.s.
Citric Acid to pH=6.5-7.0	
Sodium Chloride qs to viscosity=2000cps	
Water, Dye, Fragrance qs to	100.0

Add MACKADET BSC to water and heat to 40 degrees C. Add MACKSTAT DM. Adjust pH with citric acid and viscosity with sodium chloride. Add dye, fragrance and cool to room temperature.

#94
(Baby Conditioning)

VERNATE OP	30.0
Sodium Laureth Sulfate (30%)	14.0
VERNALENE AFC	2.5
VERNAM 35	5.0
Sodium Chloride q.s. to	2000 cps
PARAGON	q.s.
Water, Dye, Fragrance q.s. to	100.0

Add components to water and heat to 40 degrees C. Blend until clear. Adjust pH to 6.5-7.0 with citric acid. If needed, adjust viscosity with sodium chloride.

#95
(Children's Conditioning)

MACKADET BSC	25.0
MACKALENE 426	3.0
Sodium Chloride	1.5
MACKSTAT DM	q.s.
Water, dye, Fragrance qs to	100.0

Add first two components to water and heat to 40 degrees C. Blend until clear. Adjust viscosity with Sodium chloride. Add remaining components and cool.

#96

(Emulsified Baby)

1.	MACKADET BSC	30.00
2.	MACKESTER EGMS	1.50
3.	Sodium Chloride (salt)	1.00
4.	MACKSTAT DM	q.s.
5.	Fragrance, Color	q.s.
6.	Deionized Water q.s. to	100.00

Heat the water to 75 degrees C. Add #1 then #2 and start mixing slowly at 75 degrees C. until everything is in solution and is free of lumps. Keep mixing and after 15 minutes start cooling with continuous agitation cool to 35 degrees C. and add #4, #5 and mix in. Then add #3 and blend in well. If slightly higher viscosity is necessary a small amount of extra #3 can be added.

Properties:
pH 6.8 - 7.2
Viscosity 1500 - 2000 cps at 25 degrees C.

#97

(Shampoo and Rinse)

MACKAM 35HP	30.0
MACKALENE 426	5.0
POLYMER JR 30M	0.7
MACKSTAT DM	q.s.
Water, Dye, Fragrance qs to	100.0

Add MACKAM 35HP and MACKALENE 426 to water. Disperse Polymer JR 30M and heat to 60 degrees C. Stir until completely dispersed. Cool to 45 degrees C. and add remaining components.

#98

(2 In 1 Shampoo)

Ammonium Lauryl sulfate (28%)	65.0
MACKALENE 426	10.0
MACKANATE DC-30	4.0

MACKERNIUM 007	0.5
Ethylene Glycol Distearate	2.0
Sodium Chloride	0.5
Stearic Acid	0.2
MACKSTAT DM	q.s.
Water, Dye, Fragrance q.s. to	100.0

Add ammonium lauryl sulfate, MACKALENE 426, MACKANATE DC-30, Ethylene glycol distearate and Stearic Acid to water. With continuous mixing heat to 70 degrees C. and blend until homogenous. Slowly add MACKERNIUM 007 and sodium chloride. Cool to 50 degrees C. Add fragrance, MACKSTAT DM and dye. Adjust pH to 5.5-6.0 with Sodium Hydroxide if needed. Cool and fill.

Rinse

#1

(Finishing)

1.	Propylene Glycol	10.00
2.	Glycerin	8.00
3.	MACKERNIUM SDC-25	8.00
4.	Cetyl alcohol	2.00
5.	MACKAMIDE AME-100	0.50
6.	MASIL S F V	0.50
7.	MACKSTAT DM	q.s.
8.	Fragrance	q.s.
9.	Deionized Water	q.s.

Into the manufacturing tank add #9, 1,2,3,4,5 and start heating. Once the temperature is warm enough to dissolve the wax start mixing and keep heating to 75 degrees C. (170 F.). Mix well for 10 minutes then start slow cooling and reduce mixing speed to avoid aeration. At 40 degrees C. (105 F.) add #6 then #7 and use very slow mixing. Let product cool slowly and add #8 and mix in.

Properties:	
pH specs.	5.00 - 7.2

#2

(Detangling Cream)

I	SUPERPOLYSTATE®	4.00
	Cetylacohol	4.00
	AMMONYX® 4002	2.00
	ANTISTATIQUE WL 879	2.00
II	Demineralized Water	87.65
	Citric Acid	0.05
	Perfume	0.30

Heat I and II up to 80°C. While stirring, pour II into I. Cool down to 30°C and add perfume.

#3

(Cationic & Protein Conditioning)

A	VEEGUM K	1.0
	Water	39.4
	JAQUAR HP-60	1.0
B	Citric acid	0.1
	POLYPEPTIDE LSN	6.0
	Water	40.0
C	ALDO MSA	1.5
	AMMONYX 4B	7.0
	SOLULAN 98	4.0
	Preservative	q.s.

Heat water to 75°C. Slowly add VEEGUM K to the water while agitating at maximum available shear. Continue mixing until smooth. Slowly add remaining A ingredient, mixing until uniformly dispersed. Add B to A and mix until uniform. Maintain at 75°C. Heat C to 70°C and add to A/B mixing until cool.

CONSISTENCY: Flowable liquid

SUGGESTED PACKAGING: Plastic bottle.

#4

(Foaming Creme Conditioner)

Water	93.0
MONAQUAT P-TS	3.0
Cetyl alcohol (95%)	2.0
MONAQUAT ISIES	1.0
Hydroxpropyl Methylcellulose	1.0

Add hydroxpropyl methylcellulose to cold water. Stir until well dispersed, then heat to 60°C with continued stirring until clear. Add remaining ingredients and mix at 60°C until uniform. Cool to 40°C and add color, fragrance and preservative as required. Adjust pH to 4.5-5.5. Continue cooling to 25°C and fill.

#5

(Anionic Creme)

Part A	
Cetyl alcohol	3.00
Lanolin	0.50
Glycerin	1.00
Petrolatum	0.50
MACKESTER IDO	0.50
Sorbitan Palmitate	0.15
Polysorbate 80	0.15
Part B	
Sodium Sulfate	0.50
Sodium Lauryl Ether Sulfate	1.00
Animal Hydrolyzed Protein 55%	1.00
MACKAMIDE AME-75	
Hydroxy Ethyl Cellulose solution	
0.25% in water	q.s.
Butyl Cellosolve	1.00
MACKANATE DC-30	1.50
Part C	
MACKSTAT DM	q.s.
Fragrance & Color	q.s.

Melt Part A in a separate container to 75 degrees C. Into the mixing tank, add the water and add the Part B ingredients, while start the heating and mixing. Heat the contents to 75 degrees C. Then start adding the contents of container Part A slowly to the solution of Part B and using strong agitation, keep mixing for 10-20 minutes at 75 degrees C, then start cooling with agitation to 45 degrees C. Slow down agitation and add ingredients of Part C, mix very slowly, and cool to room temperature. The product will develop the viscosity of standing overnight without agitation.

Properties:
pH 4.8 - 5.4
Viscosity overnight 2500-3200

#6

(Anionic Creme)

Part A	
Cetyl Alcohol	2.20
Lanolin Anhydrous	0.25
Glycerin	1.00
Petrolatum	0.25
Part B	
Sodium Sulfate Anhydrous	0.50
MACKAMIDE AME-75	0.66
Sodium Lauryl Ether Sulfate 60%	1.00
Animal Hydrolyzed Protein 55%	1.00
MACKANATE DC-30	1.50
Part C	
MACKSTAT DM	q.s.
Fragrance & Color & Deionized Water	q.s.

Heat Part A in a separate container to 75 degrees C. Into the mixing tank put the water and then dissolve the other Part B ingredients while slowly mixing and heating the contents to 75 degrees C. Start adding the contents of container of Part A slowly to the solution of Part B, using strong agitation and keep mixing at the 75 degrees C. temperature for 10-20 minutes then start cooling with good agitation to 45 degrees C then slow agitation down and add the ingredients from Part C, mix slowly and cool to room temperature using only very slow agitation. The product will develop the viscosity overnight on standing without agitation.

Properties:

pH	4.8 - 5.4
Viscosity Overnight	1300-1600 cps

#7

(Replenishing Cream)

Water	87.60
NATROSOL 250 HHR	0.70
KESSCO ETHYLENE GLYCOL DISTEARATE	2.00
LANETTE O	2.50
MONAQUAT TG	6.70
PHOSPHOLIPID EFA	0.30
GERMABEN II	0.20

Charge water, carefully add Natrosol 250 HHR with good agitation. Heat to 50-60°C. Add next 4 ingredients and continue heating to 70°C. Cool to 45°C and adjust pH to 4.5 to 5.0. Add Germaben II. Continue cooling and agitation until pearl develops.

#8

(Cream)

CELLOSIZE POLYMER PCG-10	0.50
UCARE POLYMER JR-30M	0.50
Glycol Distearate	0.50
Cetearyl Alcohol	2.00
CETAL	0.50
PEG-100 Stearate	1.00
Stearalkonium chloride	1.70
Citric Acid	0.05
Water	92.25
GERMABEN II	1.00

Disperse UCARE Polymer JR-30M and Cellosize Polymer PCG-10 in room temperature water with agitation. Heat to 70-75°C. In a separate container add glycol distearate, cetearyl alcohol, cetyl alcohol and PEG-100 stearate and heat to 70°C. When premix is at 70°C and mixed to uniformity, slowly add it to the polymer solution. Mix until uniform. Add stearalkonium chloride and citric acid and mix until uniform. Cool to 50°C and add Germaben II. Cool to room temperature with proper mixing.

#9

(Conditioning Creme)

GLUCQUAT 100	3.0
CELLOSIZE Polymer PCG-10	0.6
PROMULGEN D	4.5
CETAL	1.2
Hydrolyzed Animal Protein	0.3
Deionized water	90.4
Perfume and preservative	q.s.

Add CELLOSIZE Polymer PCG-10 to room temperature water with propeller agitation. Heat to 75°C. When polymer is fully hydrated, dissolve GLUCQUAT 100, hydrolyzed animal protein and preservative, in that order, waiting for each ingredient to dissolve before adding the next. In a separate container, heat PROMULGEN D and CETAL to 75°C, mix, and add to batch. Mix until uniform, and cool to room temperature with adequate mixing.

#10

(Clear Conditioning)

Chitosan PCA	1.00
Olealkonium Chloride (55% Aqueous)	3.64
Water	95.36
Perfume and Preservative	q.s.

Disperse Chitosan PCA in water with high speed agitation. When completely dispersed, heat to 75°C with continued mixing until solution is clear and uniform. Add Olealkonium chloride and mix until uniform. Dissolve preservative into batch. Cool to room temperature.

#11

(Conditioning Creme)

Water	94.2
MONATERIC 1202	2.8
Stearalkonium Chloride (85%)	1.0
Cetyl Alcohol	2.0

Mix water and MONATERIC 1202 until homogeneous. Add remaining ingredients with agitation and heat to approximately 60°C. until homogeneous. Continue stirring while cooling to 25°C. Adjust pH to 4.5-5.5.

This creme rinse removes tangles for excellent wet combing and additionally provides a substantive, non-oily, non-greasy conditioning affect which leaves hair soft, shiny and vibrant.

Properties:

Appearance	Opaque Lotion
Nominal Activity	4.0%

CONDITIONER

#1

(Hot Oil)

MACKALENE 426	5.00
MACKAMIDE AME-75	7.0
POLYGLYCOL 600	5.00
Polysorbate 80	2.00
Benzyl alcohol	0.30
Dimethicone Copolycol	0.25
NATROSOL 250 HHR	0.50
MACKSTAT DM	q.s.
Water, Dye, Fragrance qs to	100.00

Disperse Natrosol 250 HHR in water. Heat to 50 degrees C. and add remaining components. Blend until clear and cool.

Properties:

Appearance:	Clear Liquid
pH:	4.4 - 4.8
Viscosity (cps, 25 degrees C):	50 - 200 cps

#2

(Hair Dressing and Scalp)

Paraffin Wax	10.2
Mineral Oil (S.G. 0.860)	35.5
Anhydrous Lanolin	12.0
MACKESTER IDO	10.0
Petrolatum	30.0
Nonoxynol-9	2.0
BHT	0.1
Fragrance	0.2

Melt all components except fragrance. Hold at 165 degrees F. Blend for one-half hour and cool to 115 degrees F. Add fragrance. Fill into containers at 110 degrees F. and allow product to set up.

#3

(Rinse-Out Gel Type With Pearlessence)

1.	Hi-Tek Polymer H 79 (Interchem Co.)	1.5
2.	Butyl Cellosolve	3.0
3.	Propylene Glycol	2.0
4.	MACKALENE 426	3.0
5.	MACKANATE DC-30	0.2
6.	MEARLMAID AA	0.1
7.	MACKSTAT DM	q.s.
8.	Fragrance and Color	q.s.
9.	Deionized Water qs to	100.0

Heat #1, #2, and #3 slowly together with #9 to 60 degrees C. Mix slowly until solution is almost clear. Then blend in #4 slowly. Mix and start cooling When cool, add the remainder.

Properties:

pH	4.2 - 4.8
Viscosity	20,000-50,000 cps

#4

(Lotion)

Oil Phase:

PROMULGEN® D	3.5
Cyclomethicone	1.0
Stearamidopropyl Dimethylamine	0.8
Dicetyldimonium Chloride (68% active)	2.0

Water Phase:

Water	91.7
GLUCAM® E-10	1.0
Citric Acid	q.s.
Perfume and Preservative	q.s.

Heat both phases to 75°C. Add water phase to oil phase at 75°C with agitation. Cool while mixing to 45°C. Adjust pH to 4-5, add perfume and continue to mix while cooling to 35°C.

#5

(Cream)

A.	Oleyl Alcohol	10.0
	MACKOL 16	2.5
	MACKESTER SP	3.0
	B H A	0.1
	Propyl Paraben	0.1
B.	MACKALENE 316	25.0
	MACKSTAT DM	q.s.
	Water, Dye, Fragrance qs to	100.0

Heat part A to 70 degrees C. Add MACKALENE 316 to water and heat to 70 degrees C. Add A to B and with continuous blending cool to 45 degrees C. Add remaining components and cool.

#6

(Clear Clean)

MACKALENE 426	6.0
MACKPRO KLP	0.5
NATROSOL 250 HHR	1.2
MACKSTAT DM	q.s.
Water, Fragrance q.s. to	100.0

Completely disperse Natrosol in cold water. Heat to 40 degrees C. and add remaining components. Blend until clear. Cool and fill.

#7
(Pearly Lotion)

MACKALENE 316	7.0
PEG 400 Distearate	0.5
Sodium Sulfate	0.5
Propylene Glycol	2.0
MACKSTAT DM	q.s.
Water, Dye, Fragrance qs to	100.0

Add first four components to water and heat to 65 degrees C. With mild agitation cool to 45 degrees C. and add remaining components. Cool and fill.

#8
(Pearl)

MACKADET LCB	10.0
Triethanol Amine	1.0
Sodium Chloride	0.5
MACKSTAT DM	q.s.
Water, Dye, Fragrance q.s. to	100.0

Warm water to 40 degrees C. Add sodium chloride and TEA. Add MACKADET LCB and blend slowly. When completely dispersed add dye, preservative and fragrance. Cool and fill.

#9
(Protein Lotion)

MACKINE 301	1.5
MACKOL 16	2.5
Lactic Acid 88%	0.7
MACKPRO NLP	1.5
Sodium Chloride	0.5
MACKSTAT DM	q.s.
Water, Fragrancee, Dye qs to	100.0

Dissolve sodium chloride in water. Add first four components and heat to 70 degrees C. Blend until homogenous. Cool to 45 degrees C. and add remaining components. Cool and fill.

#10

MACKADET CBC	5.0
MACKSTAT DM	q.s.
Water, Fragrance, Dye qs to	100.0

Add MACKADET CBC to water and heat to 70 degrees C. With continuous mixing cool to 50 degrees C. Add remaining components and cool.

#11
(High Quality)

MACKERNIUM SDC-25	10.0
MACKOL 1618	2.0
BRIJ 72	2.0
MACKSTAT DM	q.s.
Water, dye, Fragrance qs to	100.0

Add components to water and heat to 70 degrees C. With mild agitation blend until homogenous. Cool to 50 degrees C. and add dye and fragrance. Cool and fill.

#12
(With Moisturizers)

MACKOL 1618	3.0
MACKERNIUM SDC-85	3.0
Propylene glycol	1.0
Glycerin	1.0
MACKAMIDE AME-100	1.0

Mineral Oil	1.0
MACKPRO NLP	2.0
MACKSTAT DM	q.s
Deionized Water, Fragrance, Dye qs to	100.0

Melt waxes and oils to 70 degrees C. Separately heat water plus MACKPRO NLP to 70 degrees C. and add hot water solution to hot oils and waxes. Start stirring vigorously for 10 minutes then start slow cooling while mixing and at 40 degrees C. add MACKSTAT DM then fragrance and dye and slow mix down close to room temperature. Stop mixing at 30 degrees C. Adjust pH with citric acid.

Properties:	
pH	3.5 - 4.5
Viscosity (cps 25 degrees C)	1500 - 3000

#13
(Balsam)

MACKINE 301	1.6
MACKOL 16	1.8
Phosphoric Acid (85%)	0.9
Sodium chloride	0.3
MACKSTAT DM	q.s.
Balsam of Peru	q.s.
Water, dye qs to	100.0

Add the first four components to water and heat to 70 degrees C. Blend until homogenous. Cool to 45 degrees C. and add MACKSTAT DM and Balsam of Peru. Cool to room temperature and fill.

#14
(Clear Colorless Viscous)

MACKALENE 426	6.0
MACKPRO NSP	0.5
NATROSOL 250 HHR	1.2
MACKSTAT DM	q.s.

Deionized Water, Dye, Fragrance qs to	100.0

Completely dispense Natrosol in water. Add MACKLENE 426, MACKPRO NSP and blend until clear. Heat to 40 degrees C. and add remaining components.

#15
(Foaming)

MACKAM 35	10.0
MACKALENE 116	15.0
MACKPRO NLP	4.0
NATROSOL 250 HHR	0.7
MACKSTAT DM	q.s.
Water, Dye, Fragrance qs to	100.0

Thoroughly disperse the Natrosol in water and heat to 45 degrees C. Add MACKAM 35, MACKALENE 116 and MACKPRO NLP. Blend until clear. Add MACKSTAT DM, fragrance and dye. Cool and fill.

#16
(Clear)

INCROQUAT MINK-85	2.00
INCROMECTANT AQ	3.00
VOLPO 20	4.80
CROTHIX	2.10
Water	87.10
GERMABEN II	1.00

Combine the water and the Volpo 20 and heat to 65°C while mixing. Add the Crothix and continue mixing until homogeneous. Continue mixing and cool to 40°C. then add the remaining ingredients and mix until homogeneous.

#17
(Instant)

Part A

Deionized Water	81.0
INCROQUAT SDQ-25	6.0
INCROMECTANT AQ	1.0

Part B	
CROVOL A-40	0.5
VOLPO S-2	0.5
CRODACOL C-95	2.0
Mineral Oil	3.0
COSMOWAX K	2.0
CRODAMOL PTIS	1.0
Part C	
HYDROTRITICUM 2000	2.0
GERMABEN II	1.0

Combine ingredients of Part A with mixing and heat to 70-75°C. Combine ingredients of Part B with mixing and heat to 70-75°C. Add Part B to Part A with good mixing and cool to 45°C. Add Part C with mixing and cool to desired fill temperature.

Properties:
pH=
4.5
Viscosity RVT 6 @ 50rpm=5,400cps

#18
(Wheat Germ Foaming)

MACKAM 35	10.0
MACKALENE 116	8.0
MACKALENE 716	1.0
NATROSOL 250 HHR	0.7
MACKSTAT DM	q.s.
Water, Dye, Fragrance qs to	100.0

Completely hydrate Natrosol. Add first three components and heat to 40 degrees C. Blend until clear. Add remaining components and cool.

#19
(Mild Opaque)

MACKALENE 326	8.0
Cetyl Alcohol	1.8
Phosphoric Acid	0.6

Sodium Chloride	0.3
MACKSTAT DM	q.s
Water, Dye, Fragrance, qs to	100.0

Add first four components to water and heat to 70 degrees C. With stirring, cool and add dye, preservative and perfume at 40 degrees C.

#20

(Mild Pearl)

MACKALENE 326	7.0
PEG 400 Distearate	0.5
Sodium Chloride	0.5
MACKSTAT DM	q.s.
Water, Dye, Fragrance, qs to	100.0

Add the first three components to water and heat to 65 degrees C. With continuous stirring, cool to 40 degrees C. and add dye, preservative and fragrance.

#21

(Mild Salt Free)

MACKALENE 426	8.0
MACKOL 1618	4.0
MACKSTAT DM	q.s.
Dye, Fragrance, Water qs to	100.0

Add MACKALENE 426 and MACKOL 1618 to water. Heat to 65-70 degrees C. and blend until homogenous. Cool to 50 degrees C. Add MACKSTAT DM, dye, and fragrance. Cool and fill.

#22

(Natural Lipid for Professional Salon)

MACKERNIUM SDC-85	1.5
MACKALENE NLC	1.0
MACKPRO NLP	2.0

MACKOL 1618	1.8
Steareth-2	1.8
MACKSTAT DM	q.s.
Water, Fragrance, Dye qs to	100.0

Add first five components to water and heat to 70 degrees C. Cool to 45 degrees C. and add remaining components. Cool and fill.

#23

(Deep)

Part A	
Deionized Water	80.94
INCROQUAT BEHENYL TMS	6.00
INCROMECTANT LAMEA	1.00
Part B	
CROVOL A-40	0.50
VOLPO S-2	0.50
CRODACOL C-95	2.00
Mineral Oil	3.00
CROSMOWAX K	2.00
CRODAMOL PTIS	1.00
Part C	
TEA 99% (10% Soln)	0.06
Part D	
HYDROTRITICUM 2000	2.00
GERMABEN II	1.00

Combine ingredients of Part A with mixing and heat to 80-85°C. Combine ingredients of Part B with mixing and heat to 80-85°C. Add Part B to Part A with good mixing and cool to 45°C. Continue mixing and add Part C. Add Part D with mixing and cool to desired fill temperature.

Properties:
pH=
4.20
Viscosity RVT #7 @ 50rpm=6,600cps

#24

(Deep Softening)

Emulsifying Wax N.F.	6.0
Propylene Glycol	3.0
MACKERNIUM SDC-85	3.0
MACKESTER IDO	3.0
Glyceryl Monostearate	2.0
MACKALENE 426	2.0
MACKPRO NLP	1.0
MACKAMIDE AME-100	1.0
MACKSTAT DM	q.s.
Deionized Water, Fragrance qs to	100.0

Melt first five components and heat to 150 deg. F. Heat water, MACKPRO NLP and MACKAM AME-100 to 150 deg. F. Slowly add water to the oil phase and blend for 30 minutes. Add preservative and MACKSTAT DM at 110 degrees F. Cool and fill.

#25

(Spray-On For Extra Curly Hair)

MACKINE 301	1.00
MACKESTER EGMS	1.50
Cetearyl Alcohol	1.50
ALFOL 1216	1.50
Lactic Acid Natural	q.s to pH approx 0.40
Fragrance, Color	q.s.
MACKSTA DM	q.s.
MACKERNIUM 007 (OPTIONAL)	0.50
Deionized Water	q.s. to 100.00

Into the manufacturing stainless steel tank meter water, #9 and start heating. Add #2, #3, #4 and heat to 160°F (71°C) add #1, and start mixing well to dissolve all ingredients completely. Once the emulsion forms add #5 at about 140°F (60°C) and mix strongly and take a sample. Cool it and check pH and add #5 in small amounts till proper pH level is obtained. Then add Item #6, #7 and if desired #8, dissolved in a small amount of #9.

Mix to room temperature. A sprayable lotion will form upon overnight standing.

Properties:

pH	3.6 - 4,00

#26

(Leave On)

INCROMECTANT LAMEA	4.00
INCROQUAT BA 85	1.00
INCROMATE ISML	1.00
CRODAFOS SG	1.00
CROTEIN HKP SF	1.00
Silicone 190 Surfactant	.50
GERMABEN II	1.00
Water, deionized	90.50

Combine all ingredients and mix until uniform.

RECOMMENDED USE: After shampooing, towel dry hair and apply conditioner with short, quick sprays.

Properties:
pH=
3.9

#27

(Clear Leave-On)

MACKALENE 426	6.0
NATROSOL 250 HHR	1.0
MACKSTAT DM	q.s.
Deionized Water, Dye, Fragrance qs to	100.0

Completely dispense Natrosol in water. Add MACKALENE 426 and blend until clear. Heat to 40 degrees C. and add remaining components.

#28

(Spray Leave-On)

MACKPRO NLP	1.0
MACKALENE 426	3.0
MACKSTAT DM	q.s.
Water, Dye, Fragrance qs to	100.0

Add components to water. Heat to 40 degrees C. and blend until clear.

#29

(Conditioner Concentrate)

MACKERNIUM SDC-85	3.0
BRIJ 58	3.2
MACKOL 16	8.8
Peg 600 Distearate	3.0
MACKPRO NLP	2.0
MACKSTAT DM	q.s.
Water, Dye, Fragrance qs to	100.0

Melt first four components to 70 degrees C. and blend until clear. Add MACKPRO NLP to water and heat to 70 degrees C. Add oil phase to water and blend until homogenous. Adjust pH to 5.0 with lactic acid. Cool to 45 degrees C. and add remaining components.

#30

(Natural Lipid Hair Treatment and Restructurant)

MACKOL 1618	11.0
Anhydrous Lanolin	7.0
MACKANATE EL	5.0
MACKPRO NLP	2.0
MACKESTER IDO	1.0
Polysorbate 80	1.0

MACKANATE DC-30	0.6
MACKSTAT DM	q.s.
Deionized Water, Fragrance qs to	100.0

Heat oil soluble and water soluble components separately to 160 degrees F. Add oil to water with continuous mixing. Cool to 120 degrees F. Add MACKSTA DM and fragrance. Cool and fill.

#31

(Cholesterol Type Hair Treatment)

1.	MACKADET CBC	7.0
2.	Paraffin Wax	3.0
3.	MACKAMIDE PKM	1.0
4.	MACKERNIUM 007	1.5
5.	MACKSTAT-DM	q.s
6.	Cholesterol Powder	0.01
7.	Mineral Oil	1.0
8.	Fragrance, Color	q.s.
9.	Deionized Water qs to	100.0

Heat #1, #2, #3, #6 and #7 in the mixing kettle to 170 degrees C. Separately heat #9 to 170 degrees F (77 degrees C.) Start the agitation at slow, then high speed and slowly add the #9 water, keep mixing at medium speed for 15 minutes then very slowly start the cooling while mixing. At 125 degrees F (45 degrees C.) add #4 rinsing out the container with a little water and slow down the mixing and add #4, then #8 and mix till everything is completely uniform. At approximately 105 degrees F (41 degrees C) slow mixing to the lowest possible speed and when product thickens stop mixing. Check pH and apparent viscosity adjust with either a few drops of Citric acid solution or with a few drops of Triethanolamine: mix in slowly. Recheck pH.

Properties:	
pH	5.5 - 6.3
Appearance: White creamy smooth paste	
Viscosity: After 24 hours 77 degrees F (25 degrees C.)	16,000-26,000cps

#32
(Creme Hair Treatment)

1.	Paraffin Wax (MP 128 F.) 53 C.	3.00
2.	MACKADET CBC	6.00
3.	MACKESTER EGMS	2.00
4.	MACKAMIDE PKM	0.75
5.	PEG-150 Distearate	1.00
6.	MACKPRO WWP	1.00
7.	MACKERNIUM 007	1.00
8.	MACKSTAT DM	q.s.
9.	Fragrance	q.s.
10.	Deionized Water q.s. to	100.00

Into a stainless creme kettle put #1, #2, #3, #4, #5 and start heating to 75 degrees C. (167 degrees C.) Separately heat #10 to the same temperature, add it slowly with good mixing to the hot waxes in the creme kettle and increase mixing speed. Keep mixing for 15 minutes at the same temperature and speed. Then start cooling process slowly and reduce mixing speed. At 50 degrees C. (120 degrees F.) add #6, #7, #9 and finally #8. Take a sample, cool and check pH value and adjust batch if necessary, upward with a few drops of diluted Sodium Hydroxide solution or downward with Citric Acid solution. Cool batch slowly with very low speed mixing until product turns to cream.

Properties:
pH 4.00 - 6.00

#33
(Lite Creme Hair Treatment)

1.	Mineral Oil (SG 0.850)	1.50
2.	Paraffin Wax (MP 128 F)	2.50
3.	MACKADET CBC	7.00
4.	MACKESTER EGMS	2.00
5.	MACKPRO WWP	1.00
6.	MACKERNIUM 007	2.00
7.	MACKSTAT DM	q.s.
8.	Fragrance	q.s.
9.	Deionized Water q.s. to	100.00

Into stainless steel creme kettle put #1, #2, #3, #4 and start heating to 75 degrees C. (167 degrees F.). Separately heat #9 to the same temperature, add it slowly with good mixing to the hot waxes in the creme kettle and increase mixing speed. Keep mixing for 15 minutes at the same temperature and speed. Start the cooling process slowly and begin to slow down mixing speed. At 45 degrees C. (113 degrees F.) add #5 then #6, #7, #8. Check pH and adjust downward with Citric Acid solution or upwards with a few drops of diluted Sodium Hydroxide solution. Continue mixing very slowly until cool. The product will set up on standing to a soft creme.

Properties:	
pH	4.4 - 5.5

#34
(Creme Hair Treatment)

1.	MACKADET CBC	7.00
2.	Paraffin Wax	2.00
3.	MACKERNIUM 007	1.00
4.	MACKSTAT DM	q.s.
5.	Fragrance	q.s.
6.	Color	q.s.
7.	Deionized Water q.s. to	100.00

Fill the stainless steel mixing tank with the proper quantity of #7 and start heating to 160°F. start addition of #1 and then #2 and start slow mixing. Cover the tank to avoid excess evaporation. When everything is completely uniform and well dissolved so that there are no particles left stop heating. With good agitation add #3 and start cooling. Mix firmly but avoid aeration. At 120 F. start addition of #4 and when mass starts to harden add #6, if required, and finally #5 mix slowly until creme can be filled. Check pH.

Properties:	
pH	3.5 - 5.4

#35

(Mousse)

Part I	
Water	82.7
MONAQUAT P-TS	3.0
Part II	
Isopropyl Alcohol	10.0
Aminomethyl Propanol	0.3
Butyl Ester of PVM/MA Copolymer	2.0
Part III	
Dimethicone Copolyol	2.0

Mix Part I. Heat to 65°C and continue to mix until homogeneous. Cool to 40°C. Separately mix Part II at 25°C until homogeneous. Add Part II to Part I with stirring. Add Part III. Mix until homogeneous, add fragrance, coloring, or preservative as required. Cool to 25°C. Charge into aerosol container. Add propellent.

Fill:	
Concentrate	83.3
Isobutane	16.7

#36

(Natural Mousse)

Water	91.0
AVAMID 150	2.0
GAFFIX VC-713	3.0
MONAQUAT ISIES	2.0
Dimethicone Copolyol	2.0

Mix MONAQUAT ISIES and water until uniform. Add Gaffix VC-713 and mix until dissolved. Add AVAMID 150 and stir until completely blended. Add Dimethicone Copolyol and stir until homogeneous. No heat is required. Add preservative, color and perfume as required.

To Aerosolize Charge
  81.0% Mousse

19.0% Isobutane

Properties:

Physical Appearance	Stable foam
Activity	7 %

#37
(Mousse)

GLUCQUAT 100	0.25
AMEROXOL OE-20	1.00
SD Alcohol 40	15.00
Deionized water	83.75
Perfume and preservative	q.s.

Heat deionized water at 60°C and dissolve GLUCQUAT 100, AMEROXOL OE-20 and preservative into it. Cool at 40°C. Add SD Alcohol 40 to water phase and mix until uniform.

Aerosol Fill Procedure: Fill into aluminum mousse cans and charge with A-46 hydrocarbon propellant using 95% product and 5% propellant.

#38
(Soft Hold)

Part I

Water	82.85
MONAQUAT P-TS	3.00

Part II

Isopropyl Alcohol	10.00
Aminomethyl Propanol	0.15
Butyl Ester of PVM/MA Copolymer	1.00

Part III

Dimethicone Copolyol	3.00

Add MONAQUAT P-TS to water. Heat to 65°C with agitation until P-TS dissolves. Cool to 40°C. Separately mix Part II. Heat to 65°C to melt. Cool Part II to 40°C, then add to Part I with continued agitation. Add Part III. Add perfume and color as desired.

TO AEROSOLIZE:	%
Mousse F-229A	83.00
Isobutane (A-31 Aeropress)	17.00

#39

(Super Hot Oil)

Part A

1. MACKALENE 426	4.40
2. MACKAMIDE AME-75	4.40
3. POLYGLYCOL 400	4.40
4. Polysorbate 80	1.76
5. Benzyl Alcohol	0.26
6. Dimethicone Copolyol	0.22
7. NATROLSO 250 HHR	0.50
8. Tetrasodium EDTA 40%	0.15
9. Deionized Water	70.00

Part B

10. MACKERNIUM SDC-25	6.0
11. Glycerin	3.6
12. Isopropyl Alcohol	1.5
13. Butoxyethanol	0.6

Part C

14. MACKSTAT DM	q.s.
15. Fragrance	q.s.
16. Color	q.s.
17. Deionized Water	q.s.

Part A

Disperse #7 into water #9. Heat to 120 degrees F. (50 degrees C.) and add #1, #2, #3, #5, #6, #8. Blend together with appropriate mixing.

Part B

In a separate vessel blend #10, #11, #12, #13, warm slightly (110 degrees F.) to dissolve completely and clearly. Then add part B while mixing to the large manufacturing tank.

Part C
Blend #4 with fragrance #15 and add to tank. then add #14, #16 and the remainder of water #17.

Properties:

Appearance:	Clear Liquid
pH (Adjust up with Triethanolamine):	4.4 - 4.8
Viscosity (cps, 25 degrees C.):	60 - 240 cps

#40
(Curl and Oil Sheen)

Glycerine	47.0
Propylene glycol	3.0
MACKPRO NLP	4.0
MACKANATE DC-30	3.0
MACKSTAT DM	q.s.
Deionized Water qs to	100.0

Add components in order and blend until clear.

Hair Spray

#1
(Conditioning)

GLUCQUAT 100	0.25
AMERSETTE	5.00
SD Alcohol 40	74.75
A-46 Hydrocarbon Propellant	20.00

Dissolve AMERSETTE and GLUCQUAT 100 in SD Alcohol 40. Fill into aerosol hair spray cans and charge with propellant.

#2
(Non-Aerosol Finishing)

PHOSPHOLIPID EFA	0.60
SD Alcohol 40	94.10
RESYN 28-1310	3.75
Water	1.20
Aminomethyl Propanol	0.35

Add Resyn 28-1310 to alcohol slowly with adequate agitation, mix until well dispersed. Add aminomethyl propanol to neutralize, and mix until dissolved. Add remaining ingredients, color, fragrance and package.

#3

(Alcohol-Free Pump "Long Lasting Hold-Soft Natural Feel")

POLYMER ACP-1018	5.00
Water	94.70
SUTTOCIDE A, 50% SOLUTION	0.30
Fragrance, Plasticizer	q.s.

Add Polymer ACP-1018 to water. Add rest of ingredients and adjust pH to 7.0-8.0 with citric acid.

#4

(Alcohol-Free Pump "Stiff Hard-Hold Spray")

POLYMER ACO-1018	2.50
PVP/VA E735	5.00
Water	92.20
SUTTOCIDE A, 50% SOLUTION	0.30
Fragrance, Plasticizer	q.s.

Add Polymer ACP-1018 and PVP/VA W-735 to water. Add Suttocide A, fragrance and plasticizer. Adjust pH to 7.0-8.0 with citric acid.

#5

(Hair Moisturizing)

Water	94.50
INCROMECTANT LAMEA	3.00
CROSILKQUAT	1.00
INCROQUAT MINK-85	0.50
GERMABEN II	1.00

Warm water to 45°C. Add the ingredients, mixing after each addition until clear.

#6
(Pump Type)

RESYN 26-1314	6.0
MACKPRO NLP	1.0
Deionized Water	7.6
Ethanol, Fragrance qs to	100.0

Dissolve Resyn 26-1314 in alcohol. Add remaining components and blend until clear.

#7
(Comb Out and Conditioner)

Glycerin	18.0
Propylene Glycol	18.0
PEG 75 Lanolin	0.7
MACKAM CAP	0.3
MACKANATE DC-30	0.2
Disodium EDTA	0.1
MACKSTAT DM	q.s.
Deionized Water, Fragrance qs to	100.0

Add components to water and heat to 40 degrees C. Blend until clear. Adjust pH to 4.5 - 5.5 with citric acid.

Mousse

#1
(Natural Lipid)

PVP/VA E335	4.5
SDA 40 Alcohol	21.5
MACKPRO NLP	4.0
Deionized Water, Fragrance, Dye qs to	100.0

Combine components and blend until clear. Pressurize with suitable propellant.

#2
(Jojoba)

A	Water D.I.	80.0
	CELQUST H-100	0.5
B	POLAWAX A-31	1.5
	Jojoba Oil	1.0
	PVP (K-30)	1.5
C	SDA-40B (Reg)	15.2
	GLYDANT	0.2
	Perfume	0.1

Stir A till clear solution. Add B and heat and stir till dissolved. Cool and Add C ph-4.
Aerosol Fill: 85% of above concentrate
15% of A-46 Propellent

#3
(Conditioning and Styling)

Phase A

PROMULGEN® D	0.5
Water	77.0
AMEROXOL® OE-20	0.5
GLUCAM® P-10	1.0
SOLULAN® 98	2.0

Phase B

Alcohol-SDA 40	15.0
AMERSETTE®	4.0
Perfume and Preservative	q.s.

Combine phase A and heat to 75°C until uniform. Cool to 45°C and add premixed phase B. Phase B can be premixed at room temperature to avoid solvent loss. Add perfume below 40°C. Cool to room temperature and fill.

Fill:
95% Concentrate: 5% Propellant A-46

Styling Gel with Protein

Phase A	
Water	85.80
Carbomer-940	1.00
Propylene Glycol	1.00
Phase B	
Triethanolamine	1.00
Phase C	
Polyquaternium-11	2.00
PVP/VA Copolymer	4.00
Phase D	
Hydrolyzed Elastin	2.00
Phase E	
Dimethicone Copolyol	0.50
PEG-75 Lanolin Oil	0.50
Polysorbate 80	1.00
GERMABEN II	1.00
Fragrance	0.10
FD&C Green #3	0.10

Add carbomer to water with high agitation. Mix until smooth. Add rest of Phase A. Add triethanolamine and mix until clear. Add Phase C slowly, mix thoroughly. Add Phase D, mixing until uniform. Add Phase E in order and mix until homogeneous.

Sea Botanical and Herbal Hard to Hold Styling Gel

(Alcohol Free)

Phase A	
Water	81.70
Calendula Extract	0.10
Chamomile Extract	0.10

Spirulina	0.10
Allantoin	0.05
Phase B	
Polyglycerylmethacrylate (and) Propylene Glycol	0.20
Carbomer-940	0.60
SUTTOCIDE A, (50% Solution)	0.30
Triethanolamine, 85%	0.30
Phase C	
Water	10.00
PVP K-30	2.00
Phase D	
PVP/VA E735	4.00
Phase E	
PEG-60 Almond Glycerides	0.50
Fragrance	0.05

Meter water into stainless steel mixing tank. Begin heating to 50°C. Begin mixing and add rest of Phase A ingredients. Add Phase B ingredients in order given with adequate agitation to insure a homogenous mixture after each addition. Premix Phase C and add to batch. Add Phase D. Premix Phase E, add to batch and mix until uniform.

Conditioning/Styling Lotion

Water	q.s.
PVP K-90 (20% aqueous solution)	5.0
MONATERIC 1202	4.5
Hydrolyzed Animal Protein (50%)	0.5
SD-3A Alcohol	25.0
Propellent (optional)	5.0-25.0

Add ingredients in order listed, mixing until uniform between additions. Adjust pH to 4.5-5.5. Add preservative as required. If used in aerosol applications prepare as above, add to container and then add propellent.

Properties:

Appearance	Clear Liquid
Nominal Activity	3.0%

This formulation imparts both conditioning and controlled setting properties. As an aerosol mousse or a pump-on soft setting lotion the formulation can be spot applied, used as an after shampoo conditioner, or as a between shampoo revitalizing conditioner.

Alcohol Free Styling Gel

Water	83.2
Propylene Glycol	12.0
Acrylate/Steareth-20/ ACRYSOL ICS-I	2.0
GERMABEN II	1.0
Dimethicone Copolyol 193	.5
Fragrance	.5
Triethanolamine	.7
Jojoba Oil	.1

To the water add ingredients 2 thru 5 plus 7 with very slow agitation. Next add item 6 agitate till clear and package.

Setting Lotion & Conditioner

MACKALENE 316	4.0
GAFQUAT 755	8.0
MACKOL 16	0.5
MACKSTAT DM	q.s.
Water, Dye, Fragrance qs to	100.0

Completely disperse Gafquat 755 in water. Add MACKALENE 316 and MACKOL 16 and heat to 70 degrees C. Blend until completely homogenous. Cool to 45 degrees C. and add remaining components. Cool and fill.

Hair Cream

#1

A	VEEGUM	2.00

	Water	75.25
B	Propylene glycol	5.00
	Triethanolamine	1.00
C	Cosmetic Lanolin	2.00
	CARNATION WHITE MINERAL OIL	3.00
	AA CASTOR OIL USP	4.00
	GROCOR 6000 S.E.	0.75
	Isopropyl myristate	5.00
	Stearic acid xxx	2.00
	Preservative	q.s.

Slowly add VEEGUM to the water, while agitating at maximum available shear. Continue mixing until smooth. Add B to A and heat to 70°C. Heat C to 75°C. Add C to A/B and mix until cool.

Consistency: Soft cream
Suggested Packaging: Squeeze tube

#2
(Light Moisturizing)

MACKESTER TDO	15.0
Anhydrous Lanolin	3.5
White Petroleum	3.5
Castor Oil	3.0
MACKOL 1618	2.0
Polysorbate 20	2.0
Triethanolamine	0.6
CARBOPOL 940	0.6
Disodium EDTA	0.1
MACKSTAT DM	q.s.
Deionized Water, Fragrance qs to	100.0

Melt first seven components and heat to 170 degrees F. Add Disodium EDTA to water and completely disperse Carbopol 940. Slowly add oil to water phase and blend until homogenous. Add fragrance, preservative, and cool.

#3

(Light Moisturizing)

1.	Mineral Oil (SG (.850)	15.00
2.	Castor Oil	3.00
3.	Lanolin Anhydrous	3.50
4.	Petrolatum White	3.50
5.	Cetearyl alcohol	2.00
6.	Polysorbate 20	2.00
7.	Triethanolamine	0.60
8.	Carbomer 940	0.60
9.	Disodium EDTA	0.10
10.	MACKSTAT DM	q.s.
11.	Deionized Water qs to	100.00
12.	Fragrance	q.s.

Melt together #1, #2, #3, #4, #5, #6, #7 and heat to 170 degrees F.(77°C) Separately prepare a solution of #8, and #9 in the water by dispersing the carbomer with good agitation by slowly adding to the water and mixing until all lumps have dissolved. Some heating will help accelerating the process. Then heat the water phase also to 170 degrees F (77 degrees C). Slowly pour the oil phase into the water phase with thorough agitation to avoid formation of lumps. Mix thoroughly until everything is uniform. Add #10 and finally the fragrance #12. Check pH value, adjust upwards with #7.

Properties:

pH	5.3 - 6.0

Softening Gel

1.	GLUCAMATE DOE-120	3.30
2.	DEA Oleth-3 Phosphate	3.30
3.	ISOPAR L	3.30
4.	MASIL S F V	3.30
5.	Oleth-5 Special	1.66
6.	Triethanolamine	1.22
7.	MACKESTER IDO	1.66
8.	PEG-8	2.23
9.	Glycereth 26	1.66

10.	Glyceryl Isostearate	0.56
11.	Mineral Oil	1.11
12.	MACKERNIUM 007	3.30
13.	Aloe Vera Solution	37.12
14.	Deionized Water	35.00
15.	Carbomer 940	0.56
16.	Fragrance	q.s.
17.	MACKSTAT DM	q.s.

Into separate stainless steel vessel put #1-#11 and start very slowly heating to 40-45 C. (104-113 F.). (113 F.) and mix gently to obtain a clear uniform mixture. Into the main stainless steel mixing tank meter the water #14 add #13 and slowly add #15 mix thoroughly but avoid aeration. Warm the solution gently to 40-45 C. (104-113 F.) with good mixing. When all the #15 is completely dissolved add the blend #1-#11 very slowly to the main tank and mix until the product is uniform without lumps. Blend in fragrance and MACKSTAT DM at about 35 C. (95 F.). Check the pH and adjust either with #6 if too low or with a small amount of Oleic Acid.

Properties:

pH	5.8 - 7.2

Hair Care Lotion

I	Demineralized Water	63.75
	CARBOPOL ® .941	0.20
	PHYLDERM ® FILATOV AQUEUX	12.50
	LIQUIDE AMNIOTIQUE BOVIN	12.50
	Triethanolamine 99% (50% sol.) q.s. pH 6.8-7.0	0.75
II	ATELOGLYCANE®	5.00
	Demineralized Water	5.00
	Preservative	q.s.
	Water Soluble Perfume	0.30

Disperse the CARBOPOL® in water. Let stand and add the other components of Part I. Then add the T.E.A. solution in order to obtain a pH around 6.8-7.0. Then add II and the other components.

Curl Activator

#1

GLUCQUAT 100	3.00
Deionized water	32.00
UCON LB-1715	15.00
SD Alcohol 40	50.00

Dissolve GLUCQUAT 100 into water. Separately dissolve Ucon LB-1715 into SD Alcohol 40. Combine phases and mix until uniform. Package in a pump sprayer.

#2
(Gel)

Water	
Acrylate/Steareth-20/	57.7
ACRYSOL ICS-I	2.0
HYSTAR CG	10.3
Glycerine 99%	23.9
Propylene glycol	2.0
Dimethicone Copolyol 193	2.3
GERMABEN II	1.0
Triethanolamine	.7
Fragrance	q.s.
Jojoba Oil	.1

Add ingredients in descending order in a stainless steel tank, with slow agitation and mix till clear. Pack in a plastic tube or a plastic bottle.

Permanent Wave Lotion

A	VEEGUM HS	1
	Water	69
B	Cetyl alcohol	1
	CARNATION WHITE MINERAL OIL	5
	AMERCHOL L-101	5
	SOLULAN 98	2
	ARLACEL 165	3
C	Ammonium thioglycolate 60%	12
	Ammonium hydroxide	2
	Preservative	q.s.

Slowly add VEEGUM HS to the water, while agitating at maximum available shear. Continue mixing until smooth. Heat A to 80°C. Heat B to 75°C. Add B to A and mix until 35°C. Add C and mix until smooth and uniform.

Consistency: Viscous lotion.
Suggested Packaging: Opaque plastic bottle.

Hair Straightener

		Caustic	Bisulfite
A	VEEGUM HS	2	2
	Water	53	57
B	Cetyl alcohol	15	10
	Petrolatum	5	5
	CARNATION WHITE MINERAL OIL	8	5
	ARLACEL 165	5	5
C	Sodium hydroxide	2	-
	Sodium bisulfite	-	2
	Water	10	10
	Ammonium carbonate	-	4
	Preservative	q.s.	q.s.

Slowly add VEEGUM HS to the water, while agitating at maximum available shear. Continue mixing until smooth. Heat A to 80°C. Heat B to 70°C. Add B to A with rapid agitation, cooling to 35°C. Slowly dissolve C ingredients and add to A/B. Mix until smooth and uniform.

Consistency: Thick cream.
Suggested Packaging: Jar or squeeze tube.

Hairdressing & Highlighter

MACKESTER TD-88	25.0
Lanolin Anhydrous	17.0
Paraffin Wax	10.0
MACKESTER IDO	10.0
Polybutene	33.3
MACKANATE DOS-70PG	4.0
BHT	0.2
Fragrance	0.5

Melt all ingredients at 70 degrees C. Mix slowly while cooling and add fragrance at 38 degrees C. Mix in and fill into jars.

Hair Glosser

Petrolatum	27.0
Anhydrous Lanolin	19.0
MACKESTER TDO	18.0
Mineral Oil (S.G.O.850)	17.0
MACKESTER IDO	9.0
Paraffin Wax	7.0
MACKANATE DOS-70PG	2.6
Fragrance	0.3
BHT	0.1

Melt components together (165 deg. F.), except for fragrance, and blend until clear. Blend for one-half hour and cool to 115 deg. F. Add fragrance and cool to 108 deg. F. allow to set up at about 95 deg. F.

Hair Tonic

1.	MACKPRO NLP	20.0
2.	AY-166	10.70
3.	POLYGLYCOL 400	4.00
4.	Isopropyl or Ethyl alcohol	14.00
5.	Menthol Crystals	0.20
6.	Fragrance	q.s.
7.	MACKSTAT DM	q.s.
8.	D.I. Water q.s. to	100.00

Dissolve #1 in #8. Add #2 and mix to dissolve. Add #3 and mix in. Dissolve #5 in #4 and add very slowly with mixing to the batch. Add fragrance #6 and blend in. Add #7.

Properties:
pH 5.5 - 6.0
Clear Solution

Chapter III
BATH PREPARATIONS

Transparent Bath and Shower Bar

Sodium Stearate	24.0
Propylene Glycol	6.0
Glycerine	16.0
WITCONOL SE-40	11.0
Cocoamide DEA	18.0
HAMPOSYL C	10.0
Urea	3.0
Water	10.0
Monoethanolamine	2.0

Mix all ingredients except sodium stearate. Heat to 50-60°C with moderate mixing. Add sodium stearate slowly in small increments. Raise temperature to 85-90°C. Stir until clear. Stop agitation, allow all bubbles to rise to surface and pour into molds. Cool and remove.

Shower Soap

MACKANATE EL	20.0
MACKANATE OM	15.0
Sodium Lauryl Sulfate	10.0
MACKAMIDE LLM	6.0
MACKPEARL LV	3.0
MACKERNIUM 007	2.5
MACKSTAT DM	q.s.

Citric Acid qs to pH 6.0
Sodium Chloride qs to 10,000 cps
Water, Dye, Fragrance qs to 100.0

Disperse MACKERNIUM 007 in water. Add remaining component and heat to 40 degrees C. Adjust pH with citric acid. Adjust viscosity with sodium chloride. Cool and fill.

Liquid Shower Soap

Na A-Olefin Sulfonate, 40%	20.0
HAMPOSYL L-30	10.0
Cocoamide Mea	3.0
Ammonium Chloride	2.0
Water, Preservative, Color, Q.S.	100.0

Heat water and first two ingredients to 80°C, add cocoamide MEA, stir until clear. Cool to 40°C, add remaining ingredients and adjust to pH 5.0 w/citric acid.
Properties:
Lathers richly without drying the skin.

Non-Defatting Body Wash

Lauramphocarboxglycinate	35.0
Sodium Laureth (3) Sulfate, 27%	15.0
HAMPOSYL L-30	10.0
Oleth-10 Phosphate	2.0
Water, Perfume, Preservative, Etc., q.s	100.0

Mix all ingredients and adjust to pH 7.0 with HCl.
Properties:
Mild and good lathering shower liquid suitable for dry skin.

Clear Shower Gel

Sodium Lauryl Sulfate, 30%	35.0
Cocoamphocarboxpropionate, 40%	15.0
HAMPOSYL L-30	10.0

Cocoamide Mea	3.0
Water, Perfume, Preservative, q.s.	100.0

Mix all ingredients, heat to 60°C until clear. Adjust pH to 6.2 with citric acid.
Properties:
High lathering gel even on oily skin.

Clear Skin Lather Gel

Sodium Cocoyl Glutamate	40.0
HAMPOSYL L-30	10.0
Cocoamide Dea	10.0
Glycerol	5.0
Water, Perfume, Preservative, q.s.	100.0

Mix ingredients, heat to 50°C until clear. Cool.
Properties:
Spreadable transparent gel with mild lather.

High Foaming Shower Gel

Part A	
Sodium Lauryl Ether Sulfate	20.0
INCRODET TD-7C	7.0
CROSULTAINE C-50	20.0
Disodium Edta	0.1
Deionized Water	48.3
GERMABEN II	1.0
Part B	
CROTHIX	1.0
CROVOL A-70	2.0
BHT	0.1
Part C	
Perfume (BBA 860753)	0.5

Combine ingredients of Part A with mixing. Combine ingredients of Part B with mixing and heat to 65-70°C. Continue mixing and cool to 50°C. Add Part C to Part B with mixing. When clear, add Part B to Part A with mixing. Adjust pH with a 10% NaOH solution.

Properties:

pH	6.3
pH specification	6.0 to 6.5

Viscosity - 8,000cps RVT sp. #5, 20rpm, 1 min. 25°.

Bubble Bath

#1

Phase A

QUATRISOFT™ POLYMER LM-200	1.0
Water	46.5

Phase B

Sodium Myreth Sulfate (58% active)	38.0
Lauramide DEA	7.0
GLUCAM® E-20	3.5
SOLULAN® L-575	4.0
Perfume and Preservative	q.s.

Disperse the QUATRISOFT™ POLYMER LM-200 with good agitation in water at room temperature. When thoroughly dispersed, heat to 45°C with continued mixing. When a clear, uniform solution has developed, begin to add the ingredients of Phase B in the order in which they are listed, mixing moderatly after each addition. Avoid air entrapment.

#2

Water	51.0
GLUCAM® E-10	4.0
AMMONYX LO	15.0
MAPROFIX WAC	25.0
Sodium chloride, 10% in water	5.0
Perfume, preservative, color	q.s.

Add ingredients in order listed with thorough agitation, avoiding excess aeration. Viscosity can be controlled by varying sodium chloride concentration. To opacify for "creamy" appearance, add Glucate SS.

#3

	% Weight	% Active
MONAMATE LA-100	15.0	12.7
Sodium Lauryl Sulfate (28%)	35.0	9.8
MONAMID 1089	5.0	5.0
Water	45.0	-
	100.0	27.5

Mix with heat until clear. Cool. Adjust pH. This bubble bath creates large, voluminous, long lasting bubbles which do not dissipate in the presence of soap and hard water.
Properties:
Adjust pH to 6.0

#4
(Low Cost)

	% Weight	% Active
Water and Preservative	69.5	-
Sodium Chloride	0.5	-
MONAMINE 779	15.0	15.0
SULFRAMIN AOS C_{14-16}	15.0	6.0
	100.0	21.0

Mix with heat until clear. Cool. Adjust pH.

#5
(Viscous)

	% Weight	% Active
Water, preservative	23.5	-
MONAMATE OPA-30	18.5	5.5
MONATERIC CAB	33.0	10.0
Alpha Olefin Sulfonate (40%)	25.0	10.0
	100.0	25.5

Add ingredients in order listed while blending with gentle agitation. Warm, if desired, to reduce aeration.
Properties:

pH=	6.5 to 7.0

Viscosity is approx. 12,000 cps

#6
(Anhydrous Concentrate)

	% Weight	% Active
MONAMINE 779	70.0	70.0
Isopropyl Palmitate	30.0	30.0

Mix with medium agitation. Approximate viscosity 600 cps.

Bath Beads

Pentasodium triphosphate	50.0
Sodium sesquicarbonate	46.0
Perfume oil	0.5
GLUCAM® P-20	1.5
GLUCAMATE® SSE-20	1.0
SOLULAN® PB-20	1.0
Color	q.s.

Premix perfume oil, Glucam P-20, Glucamate SSE-20 and Solulan PB-20 with minimum of warming and spray onto inorganic salts mixture during dry blending process. For lightness, add Cab-O-Sil M-5. For "relaxing" label claim, add magnesium sulfate. For foaming effect, add sodium olefin sulfonate.

Bath Salts

NEWPORT BATHING SALT	90.0
Sodium sesquicarbonate	7.0
GLUCAM® P-20	1.5
Perfume oil	1.5
Color	q.s.

Premix perfume oil and GLUCAM P-20. Load half of the salt into a hopper above a twin shell blender, then add the sodium sesquicarbonate. Spray in the perfume and color solutions. Drop into blender and add remainder of salt. Blend 5 minutes only to avoid destroying crystal structure of salt. For improved emollient and foaming effects, add Solulan L-575 to color solution.

Bath Gel

#1

STANDAPOL ES-2	46.5
EMCOL 4300	25.0
MONAMID 150LW	23.0
GLUCAM® E-10	2.5
SOLULAN® 16	3.0
Perfume, preservative and color	q.s.

Premelt solid materials. Add ingredients one at a time, mixing thoroughly after each addition. Stir until uniform. For more smoothness and slip, add Solulan PB-20.

#2

STANDAPOL T	45.0
STANDAPOL AB-45	10.0
GLUCAM® E-10	2.0
Citric Acid, 10% In Water	3.0
SOLULAN® 75	3.5
MONAMID 150 LW	6.0
Water	30.5
Perfume, preservative, color	q.s.

Warm water to 45-50°C. Add Standapol T with gentle agitation. Premix remaining ingredients and warm until clear. Add with gentle agitation to water. To opacify, add Glucate SS. To impart residual silky effect, add Solulan PB-20.

#3

GLUCAM® E-10	3.0

SOLULAN® L-575	4.0
MONAMID R31-42	20.0
STANDAPOL ES-2	59.0
Water	6.0
Citric acid, 40% solution q.s. to pH 5.0-5.5	
Specially Denatured Alcohol No. 40	4.0
Perfume oil	4.0
Preservative and color	q.s.

With slow agitation, combine Glucam E-10, Solulan L-575, Monamid R31-42, Standapol ES-2 and water. Add citric acid solution to adjust pH to 5.0 to 5.5. Add alcohol and perfume oil slowly, mix until clear. For increased fragrance, increase perfume oil to total up to 8%. To increase fragrance duration, add Glucam P-20.

#4

(Clear)

	% Weight	% Active
MONATERIC CDX-38	50.0	19.0
MONAMATE CPA-40	47.4	19.0
Water	2.6	-
	100.0	38.0

Blend ingredients with gentle agitation while warming.
Properties:
at pH 7.5 viscosity is approx. 5,000 cps
at pH 6.5 viscosity is approx. 35,000 cps

Bath Gelee

#1

Sodium Laureth Sulfate (60%)	34.6
MACKAMIDE C	20.0
MACKANATE EL	45.0
MACKSTAT DM	q.s.
Dye, Fragrance, qs to	100.0

Add components in order and heat to 45 degrees C. Blend until homogenous. Adjust pH with lactic acid. Add fragrance and cool to room temperature.

#2

	% Weight	% Active
Water	23.8	-
Sodium Lauryl Sulfate (28.0%)	51.0	14.8
MONAMID 716	5.4	5.4
MONAMINE 779	14.8	14.8
Lauric Acid	5.0	5.0
	100.0	40.0

Heat water to 70°C and add ingredients in order listed with slow agitation. Pack hot. pH "as is" equals 7.7. Approximate viscosity equals 120,000 cps.

#3

(With Natural Lipid Protein)

Sodium Laureth Sulfate (60%)	20.0
MACKAMIDE CS	20.0
MACKANATE CP	20.0
MACKPRO NLP	4.0
MACKSTAT DM	q.s.
Water, Dye, Fragrance qs to	100.0

Add MACKAMIDE CS to sodium laureth sulfate and blend. Add remaining components and heat to 45 degrees C. Blend until homogenous and adjust pH to 6.5-7.0 with citric acid. Cool and fill.

#4

(With Silk Protein Quaternized
T Natural Skin Emollients)

Sodium Laureth Sulfate (60%)	20.0
MACKAMIDE CS	20.0

MACKANATE EL	20.0
MACKPRO NSP (Quaternized Silk Protein)	4.0
MACKSTAT DM	q.s.
Water, Dye, Fragrance qs to	100.0

Add MACKAMIDE CS to sodium laureth sulfate and blend. Add remaining components and heat to 45 degrees C. Blend until homogenous and adjust pH to 6.5-7.0 with citric acid. Cool and fill.

#5

(Emollient)

Sodium Laureth Sulfate (60%)	20.0
MACKAMIDE LLM	20.0
MACKANATE EL	20.0
MACKANATE WGD	10.0
MACKSTAT DM	q.s.
Water, Dye, Fragrance qs to	100.0

Add MACKAMIDE LLM to sodium laureth sulfate. Add the remaining components and heat to 45 degrees C. Blend until homogenous. Adjust pH to 6.5-7.0 with citric acid. Cool and fill.

Bath Oil

#1

Sesame Oil	28.0
Corn Oil	8.0
Mineral Oil, 70 Wt.	19.0
Decyl Oleate	16.0
STANDAMUL 1414-E	15.0
AMEROXOL® OE-2	10.0
SOLULAN® PB-20	2.0
ACETULAN®	2.0
Perfume and antioxidant	q.s.

Blend all ingredients; stir until uniform. For silky feel, replace part of oil system with PPG-36 Oleate. For added lubricity, replace part of decyl oleate with Amerlate P.

#2

AMERCHOL L-101®	10.0
Mineral Oil, 70 Wt.	60.0
ACETULAN®	2.0
MODULAN®	1.0
KESSCO PEG-100 DILAURATE	20.0
SOLULAN® PB-20	5.0
AMEROXOL® OE-2	2.0
Perfume and color	q.s.

Blend all ingredients together with slight warming. Stir until uniform. For increased water soluble emolient character, replace part of mineral oil with Glucam P-20.

#3

PROPAL	25.0
ACETULAN®	10.0
SOLULAN® PB-20	10.0
Perfume and color	55.0
	q.s

Blend all ingredients; stir until uniform. For "natural" labeling, replace part of Propal with vegetable oil.

#4

DIOL 400	30.0
PROPAL	30.0
Mineral Oil, 70 Wt.	20.0
MONAMID 716	4.0
GLUCAMATE® SSE-20	3.0
ACETULAN®	10.0
Water	3.0
Perfume and colors	q.s.

Blend all ingredients with minimum warming, stir sufficiently to mix thoroughly. Product will settle into two layers. For increased humectancy, add Glucam E-20. For increased body, add PPG-36 Oleate.

#5

Mineral Oil, 70 Wt.	77.0
ARLAMOL E	15.0
AMEROXOL® OE-2	1.0
IGEPAL CO-520	1.0
SOLULAN® PB-20	6.0
Perfume and color	q.s.

Blend all ingredients, mix until uniform. For greater dispersibility, increase concentration of Igepal CO-520. For greater lubricity, replace part of mineral oil with Amerlate P.

#6

Mineral oil, 70 wt.	62.0
ACETULAN®	7.0
Isostearyl alcohol	12.0
AMERLATE® P	5.0
PROMYR	14.0
Perfume oil	q.s.

Blend all ingredients except perfume. Stir with warming until uniform. Add perfume, stir until uniform. To lighten feel, replace part of mineral oil with Witconol APEM (Witco Chemical Co.) To add blooming effect, add Ameroxol OE-2.

#7
(Foaming)

HAMPOSYL L-30	21.0
SODIUM LAURETH SULFATE, 28%	42.0
COCOAMIDE DEA	6.0
PPG-15 STEARYL ETHER	10.0
Water, preservative, etc., q.s.	100.0

Mix all ingredients. Stir until Clear.
Properties:
The PPG-15 stearyl ether provides emollient properties to this high foaming bath additive.

#8
(Elegant Foaming)

Sodium Lauryl Sulfate	40.0
MACKANATE EL	30.0
MACKAM 35HP	5.0
MACKESTER SP	1.5
Sodium Chloride	1.0
MACKSTAT DM	q.s.
Water, Dye, Fragrance qs to	100.0

Add first four components to water and heat to 70 degrees C. Blend until EGMS is completely dispersed. Add sodium Chloride and cool to 45 degrees C. Add preservative, fragrance and dye. Cool to room temperature and fill.

Foaming Bath Liquid Creme

Part A

Sodium Laureth Sulfate (60% Active)	15.0
MACKAM 35	6.0
MACKAMIDE LLM	1.5
EMULVIS®	1.5
MACKANATE EL	0.6
MACKESTER EGMS	2.0
CHELON 40% ACTIVE	0.15
Deionized Water	25.0

Part B

CELLOSIZE QP 4400	42.0
Sodium Hexametaphosphate	2.0

Part C

Peppermint Oil (Redistilled)	1.0
Methyl Salicylate	0.5

Menthol Crystals	0.2
Polysorbate 20	2.0

Part D

MACKSTAT DM	q.s.

Heat all ingredients of Part A in a stainless steel vessel to 75 degrees C. (170 degrees F.) blend together. In separate container prepare Part B by dissolving Cellosize qp 4400 0.84% in 41.16% Deionized Cold Water, and mix until solution is completely clear and free of lumps. Dissolve item Sodium Hexametaphosphate in solution B and heat slowly to 40 degrees C. (104 degrees F.) and add whole mixture to Part A, and continue mixing. Prepare the blend of ingredients in Part C at room temperature and add to the above mixture. Mix in Part D into batch. Check pH. Filter the liquid cream through nylon gauze if necessary.

Properties:

pH	6.2 - 6.8
Viscosity	5000 - 10,000

Bath Lotion

Part A		
1.	MACKAM CAP	5.00
2.	Sodium Laureth Sulfate (60% Active)	5.00
3.	Propylene Glycol	1.00
4.	Methyl Salicylate	0.50
5.	Peppermint Oil (Redistilled)	1.00
6.	Menthol Crystals	0.20
Part B		
7.	CELLOSIZE QP 4400	1.00
8.	Deionized Water	51.60
Part C		
9.	Deionized Water	22.00
10.	CHELON 40% ACTIVE	0.40
11.	Sodium Hexametaphosphate	1.00
Part D		
12.	Sodium Styrene/Acrylates DivinylBenzene Copolymer (and) Ammonium Nonoxynol-4 Sulfate	1.00
13.	Deionized Water	10.00

Part E

14. MACKSTAT DM q.s.

Part A:	Prepare in mixing tank #1, #2, #3. And add (at room temperature) items #4, #5, #6, throughly blend together. Keep tank covered.
Part B:	In separate container prepare Part B by dissolving Cellosize qp 4400 1.00% in 51.60% Deionized Cold Water. And mix until solution is completely clear and free of lumps. Add the clear thick solution to Part A and blend together.
Part C:	In a separate container prepare the solution of #9, #10, and #11. Add to above solution.
Part D:	In separate vessel dilute #12 with #13 and mix until all particles are completely dissolved. Slowly add to above solution.
Part E:	Mix in Part E into batch. Blend together well and filter through nylon gauze if necessary. Check pH.

Properties:

pH	6.6 - 7.4
Viscosity	500 - 3000

Pearlescent Bath Lotion

Sodium Lauryl Sulfate	40.0
MACKANATE EL	30.0
MACKAM 35 HP	5.0
MACKESTER SP	1.5
Sodium Chloride	1.0
MACKSTAT DM	9.5
Water, Dye, Fragrance qs to	100.0

Add first four components to water and heat to 70 degrees C. Blend until EGMS is completely dispersed. Add sodium chloride and cool to 45 degrees C. Add preservative, fragrance and dye. Cool to room temperature and fill.

After-Bath Splash

#1

Perfume oil	2.0
GLUCAM® P-20	1.0
PPG-36 Oleate	0.6
SOLULAN® PB-20	0.6
Specially Denatured Alcohol No. 40	78.8
Water	17.0
Color	q.s.

Dissolve all ingredients (except water) in alcohol with stirring. Add water in thin stream with stirring. Age, chill and filter.

If mixture has heavy cloud or precipitate, increase alcohol and decrease water.

#2

Phase A:	
CARBOPOL 941	0.1
Water	25.9
GLUCAM® P-20	3.0
GLUCAM® E-10	2.0
Phase B:	
GLUCAMATE® SSE-20	4.0
Perfume oil	2.5
Diisopropyl adipate	1.5
Specially Denatured Alcohol No. 40	60.0
Phase C:	
Diisopropanolamine, 10% in water	1.0
Color	q.s.

Phase A: Completely disperse Carbopol 941 in water. Add Glucams with stirring. Phase B: Combine all ingredients except alcohol with stirring and just enough heat to clarify. Add slowly with stirring to alcohol. Stir until clear. Add Phase B to Phase A slowly with stirring until clear. With good mixing, add Phase C in thin stream. Mix until homogenous.

To opacify, add small amount of Glucate SS to Phase B.

#3
(Alcoholic)

S.D.A. Alcohol #40	75.0
Isopropyl Myristate	15.0
ROSS JOJOBA OIL	2.0
Fragrance	8.0

Mix all ingredients in a stainless steel vessel run through appropriate filter and package.

After Bath Deep Moisturing Lotion

Part A

PHOSPHOLIPID EFA	4.00
Steareth-21	0.40
Water	82.00

Part B

Steareth-2	1.60
Anthydrous Lanolin	1.50
Petrolatum	3.00
Octyldodecyl Myristate	2.00
Cetearyl Alcohol	4.00
Dimethicone (100_cS)	1.50

Combine ingredients in both phases separately and heat to 65°C. Homogenize (B) into (A) with continued heating until sufficiently mixed. Stir-cool to 40°C, then add fragrance, color and preservative as needed before filling.

Chapter IV

FACE & HAND CLEANERS

Mild Conditioning Facial Cleanser (Liquid)

Sodium Laureth Sulfate (1 mole EO)(25% active)	28.0
MONAMATE C-1142	12.5
MONAMID 1089	3.0
MONAQUAT P-TC	2.5
CERASYNT IP	1.5
Preservative	0.3
Water	52.2

Mix all ingredients into water stirring between additions. Heat while mixing to melt the solid materials (approx. 70°C). cool with stirring. At ∠ 40°C add perfume and colors. Adjust pH to 5.0-6.0.

Properties:

Appearance (25°C)	Pearled liquid
Nominal Activity	17%

Facial Liquid Soap

INCRONAM 30	16.00
INCROMIDE CAC	12.00
Sodium Oleate	7.50

Glycerine	16.00
GERMABEN II	1.00
H_2O Deionized	47.50

Blend all ingredients together under gentle heat. When completely uniform, continue stirring. Fill off.

Properties:	
pH	9.5±0.1

RECOMMENDED USE: Moisten face with lukewarm water. Pump liquid soap into hands, mix with water and work into a creamy lather. Massage with a gentle circular motion. Rinse thoroughly.

Facial Cleanser

#1

MACKANATE LO-SPECIAL	88.0
MACKOL 16	2.0
Brij 52	2.0
MACKSTAT DM	q.s.
Water, Fragrance qs to	100.0

Add MACKOL 16, Brij 52 and water to MACKANATE LO-SPECIAL and heat to 70 degrees C. Blend until homogenous. Adjust pH to 5.5 to 6.0 with sodium hydroxide. Cool to 50 degrees C. and add MACKSTAT DM and fragrance. Adjust solid to 40.0 ± 1.0 at this point. Cool and fill.

Properties:	
Solids, %:	40.0
pH (as is):	5.5
Appearance:	Pearly Cream

#2

(Daily)

Part A

Deionized Water	84.24
CARBOPOL 940	0.31
INCROMECTANT LAMEA	3.00

Part B

Stearic Acid	2.00
CRODAMOL PTC	1.50
Glycol distearate	1.50
CRODACOL C-70	1.50
COSMOWAX J	1.50
POLYCHOL 10	0.50
INCROCAS 30	1.00
INCROMIDE CAC	1.50

Part C

TEA (99%)	0.35

Part D

FD&C Red#4 (1% Sol'n)	0.10
GERMABEN II	1.00

Dust in the Carbopol 940 of Part A into the water with good mixing and allow to hydrate. Continue mixing, add the remaining Part A ingredients and heat to 65-70°C. Combine ingredients of Part B with mixing and heat to 65-70°C. Add Part B to Part A with good mixing and cool to 40°C. Add Part C with mixing. Continue mixing, add Part D and cool to desired fill temperature.

Properties:

pH	6.37
Viscosity RVT #7 @ 50rpm,	6000cps.

#3
(Mild)

MACKANATE LO-SPECIAL	83.0
MACKAMIDE PKM	4.0
MACKERNIUM 007	0.8
MACKSTAT DM	q.s.
Water, Fragrance qs to	100.0

Add MACKAMIDE PKM to MACKANATE LO-SPECIAL and heat to 70 degrees C. Blend until homogenous. Dissolve MACKERNIUM 007 in water and add to product. Blend until completely homogenous. Cool to 50 degrees C. with mild agitation. Add MACKSTAT DM and fragrance and cool with continous agitation.

#4

(Neutra Type)

1.	Glycerin	11.00
2.	Oleic Acid Light Grade	8.00
3.	MACKADET 40K	12.00
4.	MACKAM MLT	8.00
5.	MACKAM 35	6.00
6.	MACKAMIDE LLM	2.00
7.	Triethanolamine	3.00
8.	CHELON	0.30
9.	Sodium Hydroxide 50% Solution	0.5-1.0
10.	MACKSTAT DM	q.s.
11.	Color	q.s.
12.	Fragrance	q.s.
13.	Deionized Water	q.s.

Into the manufacturing tank add number 13 then #7 then #1, #2, #3, #4, #5, #6, #8 and start warming the mixture using low speed agitation, until everything is completely dissolved. Adjust the pH with #9 diluted with water and mix until the liquid is homogenous and crystal clear. Add more diluted Sodium Hydroxide solution, if necessary, to bring the pH upwards. Start cooling and add the remainder of the ingredients mix until cool.

Properties:
pH 8.7 - 9.3
Viscosity 5000-6000 cps.

#5

(Gel)

Water	52.1
Methyl Paraben	0.2
MONAMATE OPA-30	16.7
MONATERIC CSH-32	16.7
MONATERIC ISA-35	14.3

Add ingredients in the order listed while warming to 50°C, using slow agitation. Adjust pH while hot with phosphoric acid and pack warm. At pH 6.0 viscosity is approximately 35,000 cps. This is non-irritating to eyes and skin, offers excellent rinseability and leaves skin soft and smooth.

Face Cleansing Toner

#1

GLUCAM® P-20	5.0
Alcohol-SDA 40	35.0
Deionized Water	53.8
Witch Hazel	5.0
Acetone	1.0
Sodium Borate	0.1
Menthol, USP	0.1
Color and Preservative	q.s.

Dissolve sodium borate in water with gentle heat. Cool to room temperature and add the rest of the ingredients. Mix until clear.

#2

(Hydroalcoholic)

Deionized water	48.35
Alcohol-SD 40	48.35
Witch Hazel	2.00
Menthol, USP	0.30
BIOCARE® SA	1.00
Color and preservative	q.s.

Dissolve menthol in water with mixing. Add remaining ingredients. Mix until clear.

Body/Facial Cleanser and Shampoo

#1

(Pearlescent)

Ammonium Lauryl Sulfate (28%)	45.0
MACKALENE 426	5.0
MACKERNIUM 007	0.6
MACKAMIDE PKM	3.8
EGDS	1.0
MACKSTAT DM	q.s.
Water, Dye, Fragrance q.s. to	100.0

Dilute MAKERNIUM 007 in water and blend until dispersed. Add remaining component except MACKSTAT DM and heat to 70 degrees C. Blend until homogenous and cool to 50 degrees C. Add remaining components and adjust pH to 5.0-6.0 with citric acid.

Properties:	
pH:	5.5
Viscosity (cps, 25 degrees C.):	11.000

#2

(Clear)

Ammonium Lauryl Sulfate (28%)	25.0
MACKANATE EL	20.0
MACKAM 35HP	8.0
MACKERNIUM 007	0.5
MACKALENE 426	2.5
MACKSTAT DM	q.s.
Water, Dye, Fragrance q.s. to	100.0

Dissolve MACKERNIUM 007 in water. Add remaining components and heat to 40 degrees C. Blend until clear and adjust pH to adjust viscosity to 5,000 cps.

Properties:	
pH:	5.7
Viscosity (cps, 25 degrees C.):	6800

#3

(Pearlescent)

1. Ammonium Lauryl Sulfate 28%	45.00
2. MACKALENE 426	5.00
3. MACKERNIUM 007	0.60
4. MACKAMIDE PKM	3.00
5. Ethylene Glycol Distearate	1.00
6. MACKSTAT DM	q.s.
7. Deionized Water	100.00
8. Color, Fragrance	q.s.

Into main stainless steel mixing tank weigh in #1, #2, #4, #5, and start heating to 70°C (160°F), (and do not go above this temperature). Start mixing and keep temperature at 70° (160°F) until everything is fully dissolved. In a separate container dissolve #3 in the DI water #7 and heat to 70°C (160°F) and add this hot blend to the main mixing tank and keep mixing till solution is completely homogenous and no undissolved particles are noticable.

Start cooling while agitating well. At 50°C (120°F) add item #6 then item #8, cool to room temperature while mixing. Adjust pH if too high with a little citric acid.

Properties:
pH 5.0 - 6.00
Viscosity 1400-3000 cps.

Body Cleanser

(Pearl)

#1

Ammonium Lauryl Sulfate (28%)	60.0
MACKALENE 426	6.0
Ethylene glycol Distearate	1.0
MACKAMIDE CMA	2.0
MACKERNIUM 007	0.8
MACKSTAT DM	q.s.
Water, Dye, Fragrance qs to	100.0

Combine the first four components and heat to 70 degrees C. with continuous mixing. Dilute the MACKERNIUM 007 in the remaining water and slowly add to the blend. Blend until product is homogenous and cool to 50 degrees C. Add MACKSTAT DM, fragrance and dye. Adjust pH with citric acid to 5.0 - 6.0 and cool. If needed, add sodium chloride to increase viscosity and propylene glycol to reduce viscosity.

#2
(All Over)

	% Weight	% Active
Water, Preservative	70.7	-
MONATERIC CDX-38	26.3	10.0
MONAMID 150-GLT	3.0	3.0
	100.0	13.0

Add ingredients in the order listed and blend. No heat is necessary.

pH = 6.5 Viscosity is approx. 3000 cps.

Mild Body Cleanser and Shampoo

	% Weight	% Active
Water and preservative	53.6	-
MONATERIC 985A	21.4	7.5
MONATERIC LMAB	25.0	7.5
	100.0	15.0

Add ingredients in order listed and mix thoroughly with gentle agitation. Adjust pH level with 85% phosphoric acid. Viscosity of the shampoo increases as the pH is lowered.

at pH 7.0 Viscosity is approximately 4500 cps.

Bar Soap

#1

Soap Base 80/20	95.68
Water	1.00
Antioxidant	0.07
Perfume oil	0.75
Titanium dioxide	0.50
GLUCAM® E-20	2.00

Gently melt and warm additives to 60°C. Mix thoroughly with perfume oil. Combine and mix all other ingredients in suitable equipment until uniform. Place in soap plodder and extrude mass through heated extrusion plate. Press in usual manner to obtain finished bar.

#2

Soap Base 80/20	95.48
Water	1.00
Antioxidant	0.07
Perfume oil	0.75
Titanium dioxide	0.50
GLUCAMATE® SSE-20	2.20

Gently melt and warm additives to 60°C. Mix thoroughly with perfume oil. Combine and mix all other ingredients in suitable equipment until uniform. Place in soap plodder and extrude mass through heated extrusion plate. Press in usual manner to obtain finished bar.

#3
(Conditioning)

POLYOX WSR N-60K	0.10
GLUCAM E-10	1.00
MODULAN	1.00
Titanium Dioxide	0.50
Perfume Oil	0.75
Deionized water	1.00
Antioxidant	0.07
Soap Base 80/20	95.58

Combine and mix ingredients in suitable equipment until uniform at room temperature. MODULAN may require gentle heating in order to get optimum dispersion through soap base. Use soap plodder and extrude mass through slightly heated extrusion plate for high gloss finish. Press ribbon in usual manner to obtain finished soap bar.

#4
(Conditioning)

GLUCAM E-20 Distearate	1.50
Soap base 87/13	95.93
Deionized water	2.00
Titanium Dioxide	0.50
Antioxidant	0.07
Perfume	q.s.

Gently melt the GLUCAM E-20 Distearate. Combine and mix thoroughly with all other ingredients until uniform. Process in soap plodder, extrude and press into bars.

Syndet Beauty Bar

MONAMATE LA-100	40.0
PEG-8	20.0
PEG-75	30.0
MONAMID S	10.0

Add all ingredients and mix while heating gradually, being careful not to scorch, until melted and uniform (approx. 95°C). Pour into mold while hot. Allow to set.

Properties:

Appearance	Pale cream colored solid
pH (10% sol'n)	6.8

Cream Soap

#1
(Liquid)

A	VEEGUM	1.0
	Water	49.5
	JAGUAR HP-60	1.0

B	SIPON L22	40.0
	CRODAFOS SG	2.5
	MONAMID 716	4.0
	RITALAN	2.0
	Preservative	q.s.

Slowly add VEEGUM to the water, while agitating at maximum available shear. Continue mixing until smooth. Add the Jaguar HP-60 and mix until uniformly dispersed. Mix B well and add slowly to A. Mix until the guar gum is dissolved and composition is smooth and uniform. Avoid incorporation of air.

Properties: High viscosity soft gel.
Suggested Packaging: Plastic pump or squeeze bottle.

#2
(Emollent Detergent)

A	VEEGUM	1.0
	Water	50.1
B	Cetyl alcohol	0.3
	Stearyl alcohol	0.3
	LANACET	1.0
	NIMLESTEROL D	5.0
	Stearic acid xxx	2.0
	Cocoyl sarcosine	3.3
	PLURONIC F-68	12.0
	IGEPON AC-78	20.0
	AROMOX C/12W	2.0
C	A-C POLYETHYLENE 9A	3.0
	Preservative	q.s.

Slowly add VEEGUM to the water, while agitating at maximum available shear. Continue mixing until smooth. Heat A to 75°C. Heat B to 70°C, mixing slowly until uniform. Add B to A, mixing slowly until smooth. Add C and continue slow agitation to 45°C.

Properties:
Consistency: High viscosity cream.
Suggested Packaging: Plastic tube.

Glossy Washing Cream

A	VEEGUM	1.5
	Water	54.0
	Propylene glycol	4.0
B	ARLACEL 165	7.0
	PLURONIC F68	5.0
	MARCOL 130	25.0
	LANACET	0.5
	TRISOLAN	2.5
	Cocoyl sarcosine	0.5
	Preservative	q.s.

Slowly add VEEGUM to the water, while agitating at maximum available shear. Continue mixing until smooth. Add propylene glycol and heat A to 70°C. Heat B to 75°C. Add B to A and mix to 40°C.

Properties: Medium viscosity cream.
Suggested Packaging: Jar or squeeze tube.

Liquid Soap
#1

A	VEEGUM HS	1.0
	Water	42.0
B	Potassium hydroxide	2.0
	Water	37.5
	Propylene glycol	2.5
	Sodium lauryl sulfate 30%	6.0
C	Oleic acid	9.0
	Preservative	q.s.

Slowly add VEEGUM HS to the water, while agitating at maximum available shear. Continue mixing until smooth. Heat A to 75°C. Dissolve potassium hydroxide in water and mix in additional B ingredients. Heat B to 75°C. Add B to A and mix until uniform. Heat C to 90°C and add to A/B. Mix until cool.

Properties:
Consistency: Thin lotion.
Suggested Packaging: Liquid soap dispenser.

#2

Coconut oil soap, 40% solution	37.0
Water	25.5
Monateric ISA-35	28.5
GLUCAM® P-10	3.0
SOLULAN® 98	3.0
SOLULAN® L-575	3.0
Perfume, preservative, color	q.s.

With gentle heating and stirring, add ingredients in order listed, stirring thoroughly after each addition. Stir to uniformity with cooling. For creamy appearance, add Glucate SS. To minimize precipitation, add EDTA.

Liquid Lotion Cleanser

Water and Preservative	84.0
Opacifer E308	1.0
MONAMINE 779	15.0

Thoroughly disperse the latex polymer in the water before adding MONAMINE 779. Adjust pH to approximately 7 with phosphoric acid. Viscosity is approximately 1500 cps.

Cleansing Gel

UCARE POLYMER SR-10	0.30
POLYOX WSR N-3000 (1% AQ. SOLUTION) (PEG-14M)	5.00
GLUCAM E-20	1.00

Cocobetaine (43%)	4.45
Citric Acid	0.29
Cocamide DEA	5.00
Ammonium Lauryl Sulfate (28%)	53.57
Glycol Distearate	0.75
Deionized water	29.64
Perfume and preservative	q.s.

Add Ucare Polymer Sr-10 to water at room temperature. When well dispersed heat to 70°C. When a clear, viscous, hydrated solution is formed, add citric acid into the cocobetaine and add to Ucare Polymer SR-10 solution. Mix until uniform. Add remaining ingredients to batch at 70°C, adding individually, making certain each is uniformly mixed before adding the next. Cool to room temperature and pack.

Skin Cleanser

(liquid)

Sodium Laureth Sulfate (25%)	28.0
MONAMATE LNT-40	12.5
MONAMID 716	3.0
MONAQUAT PT-C	2.5
Water	52.7
Sodium Chloride	1.3

Blend ingredients in order listed at room temperature. Adjust pH to 6.0.

Properties:
Appearance: Clear liquid
Viscosity: Approximately 3,000 cps.

Hand & Body Cleanser

(Very Mild)

	% Weight	% Active
Water and Preservative	23.2	-
MONATERIC 951A	25.5	6.1
MONAMATE OPA-30	35.0	9.5

Alpha Olefin Sulfonate	15.3	6.1
Hexylene Glycol	1.0	—
	100.0	21.7

Add ingredients in order listed and blend. No heat will be needed. When pH is adjusted to 7.0 viscosity = approximately 6000 cps but will vary according to the AOS used.

Hand Cleaner/Shower Soap

(Pearlized)

	% Weight	% Active
Water and Preservative	29.3	-
MONATERIC 951A	20.8	5
MONAMATE LNT-40	25.0	10
SIPON LSB	17.9	5
MONAMID 1089	5.0	5
Ethylene glycol monostearate	2.0	2
	100.0	27

Add ingredients in order listed above and heat slowly to 70°C with stirring until completely melted. Cool to 40°C and adjust pH. At pH 6.8 viscosity is approximately 3000 cps.

Pearlescent Hand/Body Soap

	% Weight	% Active
Water, preservative	67.8	-
Alpha Olefin Sulfonate (40%)	22.5	9.0
Ethylene Glycol Monostearate	1.8	1.8
MONAMID 1034	1.7	1.7
MONATERIC MCB	5.0	1.5
Sodium Chloride	1.2	-
	100.0	14.0

Add ingredients in order listed while warming to 60°C. Continue agitation until EGMS has dissolved. Cool and adjust pH to level desired.

Properties: pH = 7.0 Viscosity is approx. 3000 cps.

Pearlized Lotion Hand/Body Soap

	% Weight	% Active
Water, preservative	71.4	-
Alpha Olefin Sulfonate (40%)	14.7	5.9
MONATERIC CDX-38	10.4	4.0
MONAMID 1034	2.0	2.0
Ethylene Glycol Monostearate	1.5	1.5
	100.0	13.4

Add ingredients in order listed and warm with stirring to 60°C.

Properties: pH = 7.0 Viscosity is approx. 5000 cps.

Detergent Free Hand Soap

MACKADET 40K	50.0
MACKAMIDE LLM	10.0
Sodium chloride	2.0
Tetrasodium EDTA (40%)	1.0
MACKSTAT DM	q.s.
Deionized Water Q.S. to	100.0

Add Mackadet 40K, Mackamide LLM, and EDTA to 90 percent of the water. Blend until clear. Dissolve Sodium Chloride in remaining water and slowly add to batch. Add Mackstat DM and blend until clear. If needed, sodium chloride can be increased to increase viscosity.

Hand Cleanser

#1

(Mild)

MACKANATE LO-SPECIAL	83.0
MACKAMIDE PKM	4.0
MACKERNIUM 007	0.8
MACKSTAT DM	qs
Water, Fragrance qs to	100.0

Add MACKAMIDE PKM to MACKANATE LO-SPECIAL and heat to 70 degrees C. Blend until homogenous. Dissolve MACKERNIUM 007 in water and add to product. Blend until completely homogenous. Cool to 50 degrees C. with mild agitation. Add MACKSTAT DM and fragrance and cool with continous agitation.

#2

(Cosmetic Waterless)

A	VEEGUM	2.5
	Water	67.0
	Triethanolamine	2.5
	Propylene glycol	5.0
B	Stearic acid xxx	4.0
	Cocoyl sarcosine	6.0
	Cetyl alcohol	1.0
	ATMUL 84	3.0
	CARNATION WHITE MINERAL OIL	5.0
	LANTROL	4.0
	Preservative	q.s.

Slowly add VEEGUM to the water, while agitating at maximum available shear. Continue mixing until smooth. Add remaining A ingredients and heat to 75°C. Heat B to 70°C. Add A to B mixing until smooth and uniform.

Consistency: Medium viscosity cream.
Suggested Packaging: Jar or squeeze tube.

Hand Soap

#1

(Pearlized)

Water	56.5
MONATERGE 1164	40.0
MONAMID 716	3.0
Pearlizing Agent	0.5

Mix ingredients while warming to 65 C. Agitate until uniform. Cool and adjust pH to 6.5. Add coloring, fragrance and preservative as required.

Properties:
Appearance: Off white, opaque liquid.
Viscosity: Approximately 1500 cps.

#2
(Salicylic Acid)

1.	MACKADET CA	30.0
2.	Salicylic Acid *	0.5 - 2.0
3.	MACKSTAT DM	q.s.
4.	Fragrance, Color	q.s.
5.	Deionized Water q.s. to	100.0
6.	Salt (Sodium Chloride)	q.s.
7.	Tetro Sodium EDTA 40%	0.4

Into a stainless steel mixing tank add #5, #1 and #7. Start heating to 120 degrees F. with slow mixing. Add carefully #2 and dissolve, when everything is clearly dissolved start cooling to 110 degrees F. Add #4 then #3 and dissolve, check pH and adjust upwards with diluted iron free sodium hydroxide solution to pH 6.6-7.4. Finally add small amounts of salt to bring viscosity to specification. Viscosity 800 - 2000 cps.

* Please note: Federal Register Part IV, Vol 51 Department of Health and Human Sources 21 CFR Part 348 & 358. States drug status of salicylic acid.

#3
(Triclosan)

Ammonium Lauryl Sulfate (30%)	27.0
Sodium Laureth Sulfate (30%)	24.0
MACKAMIDE LLM	6.0
Glycerine	3.0
MACKALENE 426	3.0
MACKANATE RM	2.0
Tetrasodium EDTA	0.1
IRGASAN DP 300	0.9
MACKSTAT DM	q.s.

Citric Acid to pH=	6.0-6.5
Fragrance	q.s.
Water, FD & C Yellow 5 and Red 4 q.s. to	100.0

Dissolve Triclosan in MACKAMIDE LLM. Add other components to water and heat to 45 degrees C. Blend until clear and add amide blend. Adjust pH and cool. If needed increase viscosity with amide and decrease with MACKANATE RM. Viscosity should be 5 to 10 thousand cps.

#4

(Heavy Duty Liquid)

Dodecylbenzene Sulfonic Acid	21.5
Caustic soda (50%)	5.4
Sodium Laureth Sulfate (60%)	4.0
MACKAM 35	5.5
Propylene Glycol	8.0
Water, Dye, Fragrance qs to	100.0

Add caustic soda to water and adjust pH to 7.0-8.0 with DDBSA. Add remaining components and adjust pH to 6.5 - 7.0 with citric acid. If necessary, lower viscosity with Propylene glycol, or raise viscosity with sodium chloride. Latex opacifier may be added if needed.

Properties:	
Solids, %:	30 ± 1.0
pH:	6.5 - 7.0

Pumice Hand Cleanser

#1

MACKANATE LO-SPECIAL	78.0
MACKAMIDE PKM	4.0
MACKERNIUM 007	0.5
Pumice (O 1/2 Grade)	6.0
MACKSTAT DM	q.s.
Water, Fragrance, Dye qs to	100.0

Add amide to MACKANATE LO-SPECIAL and heat to 85 degrees C. Disperse MACKERNIUM 007 in water and add to batch. Cool to 65 degrees C. and slowly disperse pumice. With continuous mixing add MACKSTAT DM and fragrance at 45 degrees C. Continue to mix with cooling and fill at 35 degrees C.

#2

MACKANATE LO-SPECIAL	78.5
MACKAMIDE PKM	4.0
MACKERNIUM 007	0.8
Pumice (Grade 0 1/2)	6.0
MACKSTAT DM	q.s.
Water, Fragrance qs to	100.0

Add MACKAMIDE PKM to MACKANATE LO-SPECIAL and heat to 70 degrees C. Blend until homogenous. Dissolve MACKERNIUM 007 in water and add to product. Blend until completely homogenous. Slowly add pumice until completely dispersed. Cool to 50 degrees C. with mild agitation. Add MACKSTAT DM and fragrance and cool with continous agitation.

Germicidal Hand Cleanser

MACKANATE LO-SPECIAL	83.0
MACKAMIDE PKM	4.0
Choroxylenol	0.5
MACKERNIUM 007	0.8
MACKSTAT DM	q.s.
Water, Fragrance qs to	100.0

Add MACKAMIDE PKM and Choroxylenol to MACKANATE LO-SPECIAL and heat to 70 degrees C. Blend until homogenous. Dissolve MACKERNIUM 007 in water and add to product. Blend until completely homogenous. Cool to 50 degrees C. with mild agitation. Add MACKSTAT DM and fragrance and cool with continous agitation.

Hand Safety Cleaner

1.	MACKADET SBC-8	40.00
2.	MORTON THIOKOL #295	1.20
3.	Sodium chloride	0.75-1.00
4.	Fragrance	q.s.

5.	MACKSTAT DM	q.s.
6.	Deionized Water	q.s.
7.	Color	q.s.

Dissolve #1 and #5 in 3/4 of water (#6) with good mixing, make sure everything is completely dissolved. Dissolve #3 in part of the remaining water (#6) and mix everything well. Separately blend #2 with the rest of the available water (#6) until completely in solution. Add this solution very slowly to the tank while mixing. Add #4 and finally #7 if required. Adjust pH if necessary with citric acid or dilute sodium hydroxide solution and viscosity with salt solution. Filter product if necessary.

Properties:

pH	6.5-7.00
Viscosity	5000-10,000 cps

Gel Waterless Hand Cleaner

#1

Water	58.0
MONAMINE 853	11.0
Deodorized Kerosene	27.0
Oleic Acid	4.0

Add ingredients in the order listed with good agitation.

#2

(Slow Setting)

The addition of Gafac RM-510 to the basic formulation delays the set-time sufficiently to permit liquid filling of containers, and eliminates the need for heavy mixing and piston filling equipment. This system remains flowable for approximately one hour after filling, and on standing overnight develops the desired "pinging" gel structure.

Water	58.0
MONAMINE 853	11.0
GAFAC RM-510	2.0
Deodorized Kerosene	27.0
Oleic Acid	2.0

Add ingredients in the order listed with good agitation.

Hand Cleaner For Wall Dispenser

	% Weight	% Active
Water, preservative	62.0	-
MONAMATE OPA-30	15.0	4.5
MONATERIC LMM-30	15.0	4.5
Sodium Lauryl Ether Sulfate (25%)	8.0	2.0
TOLUTRIAZOLE	q.s.	-
	100.0	11.0

Add ingredients in order listed and blend until homogenous.

Properties:
pH = 5.8 Viscosity is approx.. 300 cps

Chapter V

MAKEUP

Moisturizing Make-Up Foundation

Part A

PHOSPHOLIPID EFA	3.00
0.5% Kelzan AR in 1.0% NaCl	72.50
Pigment	15.00
Steareth-20	1.60
Methyl Paraben	0.25

Part B

Isopropyl Myristate	2.00
Hexyl Laurate	2.00
Steareth-2	2.40
Dimethylpolysiloxane (200cS)	1.00
Propyl Paraben	0.25

Combine ingredients in both phases separately and heat to 65°C. Homogenize Part A thoroughly. Add (B) to (A) and continue to homogenize. Stir-cool, with minimal aeration, to 40°C, then fill.

Anhydrous Cream Makeup

AMERCHOL® RC	5.0
MODULAN®	5.0
SOLULAN® PB-2	5.0
Petrolatum	40.0

Mineral Oil, 70 vis.	22.0
Microcrystalline Wax, (190-195°F m.p.)	8.0
Pigments, micronized	15.0
Perume and Preservative	q.s.

Heat all ingredients except the pigment blend to 85°C. Add the pigment blend to melted wax phase at 85°C. Mix until uniform. Cool to 60°C and pour.

Emulsion Makeup

Oil Phase	
AMERCHOL L-101®	4.5
AMERLATE® P	0.9
Stearic Acid, XXX	2.7
Glyceryl Monostearate, neut.	1.8
Mineral Oil, 70 vis.	4.5
Water Phase	
Propylene Glycol	4.5
Triethanolamine	0.9
Water	70.2
Titanium Dioxide, Talc & Pigments	10.0
Perfume and Preservative	q.s.

Add the water phase at 85°C to the oil phase at 95°C while stirring. Continue mixing, and cool to 30°C. Add to the micronized powder blend in increments, mixing well after each addition.

Fluid Make-Up

I	HYDROLACTOL® .70	12.00
	Cety Alcohol	2.00
	M.O.D. WL 2949	3.00
	D.P.P.G.	4.00
	MINERAL OIL	4.00
A	BROWN PIGMENTS (Cl 77492-77491-77499)	1.15
	LABRAFIL ® ISOSTEARIQUE	0.50
B	YELLOW PIGMENT (CI77 491)	0.35

	LABRAFIL ® ISOSTEARIQUE	0.20
C	LIPOPHILIC TITANIUM DIOXYDE	4.50
	LABRAFIL ® ISOSTEARIQUE	1.00
II	Demineralized Water	60.00
	BLANOSE ® CMC 7 LFD	1.00
	VEEGUM ® HV	1.00
	Preservative	q.s.
	S.A.B.	5.00
	Perfume	0.30

Prepare A, B and C by using a three-roll mill (3 times). Disperse the BLANOSE ® and the VEEGUM ® in demineralized water. Heat I and II up to 75°C and mix well the dispersion of pigments in I by using a high speed stirrer. Pour II at 75°C into I at 75°C. Stir using normal conditions. Cool down and around 30°C, add the other components. Mix weel until homogeneous.

Pressed Powder Blush

I	Kaolin	2.00
	ORGASOL ® 2002 D. NAT. COS. EXTRA	6.00
	Talcum	60.30
	PRECIROL ® ATO 5	3.00
	Magnesium Carbonate	1.00
	Lipophilic Titanium Dioxyde	10.50
	Methyl Paraben, Sodium Salt	0.20
II	ISOSTEARATE D'ISOSTEARYLE	6.00
	LABRAFIL ® ISOSTEARIQUE	2.00
	Iron Oxyde Red N° 27 (CI 77491)	5.40
	F D C Red 3 Aluminium Lake (CI 45430 : 1)	3.60

Mix well together the components of I. Add II and the pigments. Mix well and grind. Sift. Compact at 100 kg of pressure.

Cream Rouge

Part A

ROSS REFINED #1 YELLOW CARNAUBA WAX	6.0
ROSS OZOKERITE WAX 77W	10.0
Mineral Oil	24.0
Isopropyl Palmitate	27.0

Part B

Talc	10.0
Titanium Dioxide	20.0
Color	3.0

Melt Part A to 70.C. When cooled run together with Part B on the three roll mill.

Moisture Stick Base

Mineral Oil 80/90 Visc.	47.0
ROSS WAX 26-1152	28.0
ROSS WAX 15-1182	2.0
ROSS WAX 1824	10.0
Jojoba Oil	2.0
AMERLATE P	10.0
Vitamin E	1.0

Melt all ingredients together in a kettle to 170.F under agitation. When mixed thoroughly pour into molds. Capping may be necessary.

Lipstick

#1

I	APIFIL®	2.13
	Phenyldimethicone	2.13
	Mineral Wax	23.15
	ISOSTEARATE D'ISOSTEARYLE	31.57
	D.P.P.G.	3.20
	HYDROPHILOL ® ISOSTEARIQUE	2.13
	LIPOCIRE ® A	4.26
	Cetyl Lactate	1.78
	LAFIL ®	4.45
	Castor Oil	14.25
	Antioxygen	q.s.

II	LABRAFIL ® ISOSTEARIQUE	6.00
	F.D.C. Yellow 5 AL. Lake (CI 19140:1)	2.00
	D.C. Red 7 CA (CI 15850:1)	1.00
	Lipophilic Titanium Dioxyde	1.65
	Perfume	0.30

Mix all the components of II well and pass this mixture through a three roll mill (three times). Heat I at 75-80°C. Mix well. With a slow stirring, pour II into I and add the perfume. Mix well until good homogeneity. Maintain the temperature at 70-75°C and pour into molds.

#2

ROSS SYNTHETIC CANDELILLA WAX	11.2
Isopropyl Myristate	9.8
Lanolin N.F.	4.5
ROSS WHITE BEESWAX N.F.	3.4
ROSS REFINED PARAFFIN WAX 130/35	2.1
ROSS WHITE OZOKERITE WAX 77W	1.0
Castor Oil	55.6
Pigment	12.3
Teg. "P"	0.1
	100.0

Melt all ingredients and mix together thoroughly. Cool to 70°C and mold. Lipstick components should not be heated in excess of 80°C.

#3
(High Shine)

Castor Oil	59.4
Candelilla Wax	8.0
ACETULAN	7.5
ROSS WAX 1275W	5.0
Propylene Glycol Monolaureate	5.0
LANOGENE	5.0
Carnauba Wax	2.0
Propylparaben	0.1
TIMIRON MP-10	7.0
D & C Red #7 CA Lake (13107)	0.9
Pur. Navy Blue #7110	0.1

Fragrance	q.s.

Grind the pigments in part of the Castor Oil using either a 3-roll mill or mortar/pestle. Add all other ingredients (except for pearlscent pigment and fragrance) and heat gently on steam bath to 80-85.C. Add pearl, mix until homogeneous. Fragrance should be added at lowest possible temperature. Cast into molds.

Lip Balm

#1

GLUCAM E-20 Distearate	5.0
Candelila wax	30.0
Castor oil	65.0

Heat gently to 75°C with mixing until homogeneous. Cast into molds.

#2

(Protective)

Shea Butter (and) Beeswax (and) Candelilla Wax	56.00
Petrolatum	33.00
Ceresin	5.00
Calendula Extract	2.00
Candelilla Wax	0.50
Tocopheryl Acetate (Vitamin E Acetate)	2.00
Benzophenone-3 (Oxybenzone)	1.00
Allantoin	0.50

Weigh all ingredients, except calendula extract, and heat with mixing until melted. Cool to 50°C and add calendula. Mix and pour into containers.

#3

CASTOR OIL CRYSTAL O	46.0
EMERY IPP	17.0
EMERY 1723	10.4
ROSSWAX 2640	19.6

Acetulan	2.5
SDA Alcohol #40	2.0
SOLAR CHEM O	1.5
Propylene Glycol	1.0
Fragrance GP-58	q.s.

Melt all ingredients to 190.F in a stainless steel vessel. Mix throughly with agitation. Cool to 165.F, add fragrance and pour into a container. Note: Capping may be necessary.

#4

ROSS BASE OIL 2539	55.4
EMERY 1723	10.8
ROSSWAX 2611	29.3
SPA Alcohol = 10	2.0
SOLAR CHEM O	1.5
Propylene Glycol	1.0
Fragrance GP-58	q.s.

Melt all ingredients to 190.F in a stainless steel vessel. Mix throughly with agitaiton. Cool to 165.F, add fragrance and pour into a container. Note: Capping may be necessary.

#5
(White)

	%
ROSSWAX 2639	85.0
Mineral Oil #7	13.5
SOLAR CHEM O	1.5
Fragrance GP-58	q.s.

Melt all ingredients to 190.F in a stainless steel vessel. Mix throughly with agitation, cool to 165.F, add fragrance and pour into a container. Note: Capping may be necessary.

Mascara

I	APIFIL ®	8.00
	COMPRITOL ® 888 ATO	1.50
	Castor Oil	2.00
II	Demineralized Water	53.60

	CARBOPOL ® .934	0.30
	Triethanolamine 99% (50% Sol.)	0.60
	Preservative	q.s.
III	Iron Oxyde Black N° 16 (CI 77499)	7.00
	Talcum	10.00
	LABRAFIL ® .ISOSTEARIQUE	10.00
	COPOLYMER 845	7.00

Disperse the CARBOPOL ® in demineralized water. Let stand. Heat I and II at 75°C. Under stirring, pour II at 75°C. Add the T.E.A. solution and preservative. Maintain stirring while cooling. At about 30-35°C, add III and the COPOLYMER. Maintain stirring until homogeneous. (Part III will be prepared using a three roll mill - 3 times.)

Pot Eyeshadow

Mineral Oil 70/80	40.0
Petrolatum	15.0
ROSS OZOKERITE WAX 77W	20.0
ROSS REFINED CANDELILLA LIGHT FLAKES 4.0	
Pigment Paste	20.0
Preservative	1.0

Grind color with oil and petrolatum in roller mill. Heat waxes until melted and add pigment paste. Maintain 85 C for 30 minutes with agitation. Pour into molds.

Clear Eye Gel

Deionized water	57.75
Carbomer 940 (3% aqueous slurry)	25.00
Triethanolamine (10% aqueous solution)	11.25
GLUCAM ® E-10	5.00
BioCare ® SA	1.00
Perfume and preservative	q.s.

Add carbomer 940 slurry to water with gentle agitation; when fully dissolved mix in remaining ingredients, triethanolamine last. Slowly mix to avoid air entrapment until gel is formed.

Make-Up Remover

#1

MACKANATE CP	35.0
MACKANATE UM	5.0
MACKSTAT DM	q.s.
Water, Fragrance, Dye qs to	100.0

Add components to water and heat to 40 degrees C. Blend until clear.

#2

(Liquifying Cream)

PENRECO MINERAL OIL #9	51.08
PETROLATUM ALBA	32.80
ROSSWAX 60-0254	9.10
ROSS CERESINE WAX 1160/7	7.00
Beta Carotene 30%	0.02
Fragrance	q.s.
Preservative	q.s.

Melt ingredients one thru four in a steam jacketed kettle to 170. F with good agitation. When fully mixed cool, add the rest of the ingredients and pack at about 130. F.

#3

(Lotion)

I	TEFOSE ® .2000	7.00
	Cetyl alcohol	2.00
	ISOSTEARATE D'ISOSTEARYLE	8.00
	M.O.D. WL 2949	5.00
II	Demineralized Water	77.50
	CARBOPOL ® 941	0.10
	Triethanolamine 99% (50% solution)	0.20
	Preservative	q.s.
	Perfume	0.20

Disperse the CARBOPOL ®. Let stand. Under stirring, pour II heated up to 75°C into I heated up to 75°C. Add the Triethanolamine solution. Cool down while stirring and around 35°C, add the other components.

Oil Free Eye Makeup Remover

GLUCAM® P-10	2.7
GLUCAMATE® SSE-20	2.0
Boric Acid	0.3
Cocoamphocarboxglycinate (and) Sodium Trideceth Sulfate (and) Hexylene Glycol	5.0
Deionized Water	90.0
Preservative	q.s.

Dissolve GLUCAMATE® SSE-20 and boric acid in water by gentle heating to 60°C. Add the rest of the ingredients. Mix until clear.

Chapter VI

CREAMS & LOTIONS

All-Purpose Cream

#1

(Soft Texture)

Oil Phase

GLUCATE® SS	0.8
ACETULAN®	1.0
Peanut oil	12.0
Glyceryl monostearate, neut.	5.0
SPERMWAX	4.0

Water Phase

GLUCAMATE® SSE-20	1.2
GLUCAM® E-20	5.0
Water	71.0
Perfume and Preservative	q.s.

Add the water phase at 85°C to the oil phase at 85°C while mixing. Continue mixing while cooling to 50°C. Add perfume. Stir to 35°C. Homogenize and pack To vary natural base, replace peanut oil with other liquid vegetable oils.

#2

Oil Phase	
AMERCHOL® 400	3.00
SOLULAN® 25	1.00
Mineral oil, 70 vis.	16.50
Petrolatum, USP white	3.00
Water Phase	
CARBOPOL 934	0.75
Water	68.25
Triethanolamine, 10% aq.	7.50
Perfume and Preservative	q.s.

Disperse the Carbopol in the water using high speed mixing. Heat to 65°C. Add to the oil phase at 65°C while mixing. When the emulsion has formed, add the triethanolamine solution. Continue mixing and cool to 45°C. Add perfume. Stir to 30°C. To reduce oiliness, replace part of mineral oil with ACETULAN. For satiny feel, replace part of mineral oil with PPG-36 Oleate. For better emulsification, replace petrolatum with AMERCHOL 400.

#3
(Light)

Oil Phase	
AMERCHOL L-101®	5.0
MODULAN®	2.0
Glyceryl monostearate, neut.	7.0
Myristyl myristate	2.0
Mineral oil, 70 vis.	4.0
Silicone 200 fluid, 350 cstks.	0.5
Water Phase	
Sorbitol, 70%	5.0
ALBAGEL	1.5
TRITON X-400	1.0

Water	72.0
Perfume and Preservative	q.s.

Disperse Albagel in water at 80°C with high speed mixing. Add water phase to oil phase while stirring at 80°C. cool and stir to 50°C. Add perfume. Stir to 35°C. To reduce tackiness, replace sorbitol with GLUCAM E-20.

#4

(Emollients)

Oil Phase

GLUCATE® SS	0.8
MODULAN®	2.0
Cetyl alcohol	2.0
Mineral oil, 70 vis.	6.0
Stearic acid	2.0

Water Phase

GLUCAMATE® SSE-20	1.2
GLUCAM® E-20	5.0
ALBAGEL	1.5
Water	79.5
Perfume and Preservative	q.s.

Disperse the Albagel thoroughly in the water using high speed mixing. Add the Glucamate SSE-20 and heat while mixing. Add the water phase at 80°C to the oil phase at 80°C. Continue mixing while cooling to 45°C, add perfume, mix to 35°C. Homogenize and pack.

To increase viscosity, replace part of cetyl alcohol with stearyl alcohol. For tube packaging, replace cetyl alcohol with myristyl alcohol. For reduced oilness, replace part of mineral oil with ACETULAN.

#5
(Firm)

Oil Phase

AMERCHOL L-101®	6.0
ACETULAN®	2.0
Silicone fluid 200, 350 cstks.	1.0
Stearic acid, xxx	5.0
Cetyl alcohol	2.0
Glyceryl monostearate, neut.	5.0
SPERMWAX	5.0

Water Phase

Triethanolamine	1.0
Propylene glycol	4.0
Water	69.0
Perfume and Preservative	q.s.

Add water phase to oil phase at 85°C with good stirring. Stir and cool to 45°C. Add perfume, stir to 30°C.

For improved lubricity, replace part of stearic acid with AMERLATE LFA. For satiny feel, replace part of Spermwax with PPG-36 Oleate. For reduced tackiness, replace propylene glycol with GLUCAM E-10.

#6
(Silicone-liquid)

Oil Phase

AMERCHOL L-101®	5.0
ACETULAN®	3.0
Glyceryl monostearate, s.e.	10.0
Cetyl alcohol	2.0
Silicone fluid 200, 350 cstkks.	10.0

Water Phase

PVP K-30	2.0
Sodium lauryl sulfate	0.4
Water	67.6
Perfume and Preservative	q.s.

Heat water to 90°C, dissolve PVP K-30 thoroughly while stirring. Add sodium lauryl sulfate. Add water phase at 90°C to oil phase at 85°C with good stirring. Cool and stir to 45°C. Add perfume, stir to 32°C. Homogenize. For less tackiness, replace PVP K-30 with GLUCAM E-10. For higher viscosity, replace part of cetyl alcohol with stearyl alcohol. For lower viscosity, replace part of cetyl alcohol with myristyl alcohol.

#7

(Pearlescent)

Oil Phase

AMERCHOL L-101®	5.0
SOLULAN® 16	3.0
Silicone fluid 200, 350 cstks.	1.0
Myristyl myristate	5.0
Cetyl alcohol	10.0

Water Phase

Glycerine	2.5
Water	73.4
HYAMINE 10X	0.1
Perfume and Preservative	q.s.

Add the water phase at 85°C to the oil phase at 85°C while mixing. Continue mixing while cooling to 45°C, add perfume and cool to 30°C.

To add cationic (substantive to protein) properties to this formula, increase Hyamine 10X concentration to 1.0%. For less tacky, residual feel, replace glycerine with GLUCAM E-20. To increase viscosity, replace part of cetyl alcohol with stearyl alcohol. To decrease viscosity, replace part of cetyl alcohol with myristyl alcohol.

#8
(Coconut Oil Base)

Oil Phase

SOLULAN® 5	1.0
Coconut oil	10.0
Stearic acid, xxx	4.0
SPERMWAX	3.0
Glyceryl monostearate, s.e.	5.0
Cetyl alcohol	1.0
Silicone fluid 200, 350 cstks.	2.0

Water Phase

Triethanolamine	1.5
Sorbitol solution, 70%	4.0
Water	68.5
Perfume and Preservative	q.s.

Add the water phase at 85°C to the oil phase at 85°C while mixing. Continue mixing while cooling to 45°C. Add perfume. Stir to 30°C.

For lubricity, replace silicone fluid with AMERLATE P. For greater firmness, replace cetyl alcohol with stearyl alcohol. For complete rub-in, replace sorbitol with GLUCAM E-20.

#9
(Hand & Body)

Oil Phase

AMERCHOL® CAB	10.0
MODULAN®	2.0
Glyceryl monostearate, neut.	6.0
Cetyl alcohol	2.0
Mineral oil, 70 vis.	6.0
Myristyl myristate	4.0
Stearic acid, xxx	5.0
Silicone 200 fluid, 350 cstks.	0.5

Water Phase

Glycerine	4.0
Sodium lauryl sulfate	0.5
Water	60.0
Perfume and Preservative	q.s.

Add water phase to oil phase at 80°C with good stirring. Cool while stirring to 50°C. Add perfume. Stir to 37°C.

For firmer consistency, replace part of cetyl alcohol with stearyl alcohol. For less residual feel and a feeling of dry film, replace glycerine with GLUCAM E-20. For lighter texture, replace stearic acid with AMERLATE LFA.

Cleansing Cream

#1

Oil Phase

OHlan	3.0
Amerlate P	2.0
Beeswax	10.0
Mineral Oil, 80-90 vis.	44.0
Glyceryl Stearate	2.0
Ozokerite	5.0

Water Phase

Borax	0.6
Water	28.6
BIOCARE POLYMER HA-24	3.8
GERMABEN® IIE	1.0

Add BioCare Polymer HA-24 to water at 25°C. Mix until thoroughly dispersed. Heat to 45-50°C if necessary. When dispersed, add Borax and heat to 80°C. Add water phase to the oil phase at 80°C while mixing. Add Germaben IIE at 75°C. Continue to mix until 35°C.

#2
(Enriched Glossy)

Oil Phase

AMERCHOL L-101®	3.0
AMERLATE® P	1.0
Beeswax, USP	17.0
Mineral oil, 70 vis.	21.5
Isopropyl palmitate	21.5
Glyceryl monostearate, neut.	2.0

Water Phase

Borax, USP	1.0
Water	33.0
Perfume and Preservative	q.s.

Add water phase to oil phase at 75°C with good mixing. Cool while stirring to 45°C. Add perfume, stir to 30°C.

#3
(Soap Free)

Oil Phase

AMERCHOL L-101®	3.0
Beeswax, U.S.P.	4.0
Paraffin, 133°F m.p.	5.3
Cetyl alcohol	1.0
Ceresin	2.7
Mineral oil, 70 vis.	20.0
Silicone fluid 200, 350 cstks.	1.0
Sorbitan monostearate	2.0

Water Phase

SOLULAN® 25	2.0
Polysorbate 60	4.0
CARBOPOL 940	0.4

Triethanolamine (10% aq.)	4.0
Water	50.6
Perfume and Preservative	q.s.

Dissolve the Polysorbate 60 and Solulan 25 in the water. Disperse the Carbopol 940 in the polysorbate 60 and Solulan 25 solution using high speed mixing. Mix until free from lumps. Add the oil phase at 85°C to the water phase at 85°C while mixing. After the emulsion has formed and when the temperature drops to 60°C, add the triethanolamine solution. Continue mixing and cool to 45°C, add perfume, cool to 35°C.

#4

(Rinsable)

Oil Phase

AMERCHOL L-101®	3.0
ACETULAN®	4.0
Beeswax, USP	10.0
Ozokerite	7.0
Glyceryl monostearate, s.e.	2.0
Mineral oil, 70 vis.	30.0

Water Phase

Borax, USP	0.60
Triethanolamine	0.25
Water	43.15
Perfume and Preservative	q.s.

Add water phase to oil phase at 75°C with good stirring. Stir and cool to 45°C. Add perfume, stir to 30°C.

#5

(Rinse-off)

Oil Phase

AMERLATE® p	3.0
STANDAMUL 1414E	5.0
Isopropyl myristate	8.0

Cetyl alcohol	8.0
CERAPHYL 140-a	3.0
CERASYNT SD	4.5

Water Phase

GLUCAM-20	5.0
Water	58.5
Propylene glycol	2.0
STANDAPOL SHC 101	3.0
Perfume and Preservative	q.s.

Heat both phases to 75°C. Add water phase to oil phase while stirring. Allow to cool with continued agitation to 45°C. Add fragrance, stir to 38°C.

For softer consistency, replace part of cetyl alcohol with myristyl alcohol. For firmer consistency, replace part of cetyl alcohol with stearyl alcohol.

#6
(Washable)

Oil Phase

SOLULAN® 75	2.0
SONOJELL #9	7.5
TWEEN 60	1.0
Cetyl alcohol	7.0
CERASYNT SE	7.0
Isopropyl myristate	7.5

Water Phase

GLUCAM® E-20	2.5
Water	63.0
Propylene glycol	2.5
Perfume and Preservative	q.s.

Heat both phases to 75°C. Add water phase to oil phase while stirring. Allow to cool with continued agitation to 45°C. Add perfume, stir to 38°C.

For softer, glossier consistency and appearance, replace part of Sonojell with AMERCHOL CAB. For firmer consistency, replace part of cetyl alcohol with stearyl alcohol.

#7

(Pearlescent)

MACKANATE LO-SPECIAL	83.0
MACKAMIDE PKM	4.0
Stearic Acid	0.3
MACKERNIUM 007	0.8
MACKSTAT DM	q.s.
Water, Fragrance qs to	100.0

Add MACKAMIDE PKM to MACKANATE LO-SPECIAL and heat to 70 degrees C. Blend until homogenous. Dissolve MACKERNIUM 007 in water and add to product. Blend until completely homogenous. Cool to 50 degrees C. with mild agitation. Add MACKSTAT DM and fragrance and cool with continous agitation.

#8

(Cleansing W/O Cream)

A	VEEGUM	2
	Water	37
B	CARNATION WHITE MINERAL OIL	20
	Petrolatum	9
	Isopropyl myristate	5
	LANTROL	3
	Sorbitol 70%	20
	ARLACEL 186	3
	TWEEN 80	1
	Preservative	q.s.

Slowly add VEEGUM to the water, while agitating at maximum available shear. Continue mixing until smooth. Heat A to 70-75°C. Heat B to 70-75°C. Add A to B with high shear mixing. Mix until room temperature is reached.

Consistency: Soft cream.
Suggested Packaging: Pump or squeeze bottle.
Comments: When used as a cleansing cream, apply to the face and throat with fingertips. Remove with a tissue or soft cloth.

#9
(Heavy Duty W/O)

Oil Phase

OHlan™	3.0
AMERLATE® P	2.0
Beeswax, USP	10.0
Mineral oil, 80-90 vis.	44.0
Glyceryl monostearate, neut.	2.0
Ozokerite	5.0

Water Phase

Borax, USP	0.6
Water	33.4
Perfume and Preservative	q.s.

Add the water phase at 80°C to the oil phase at 80°C while mixing. Continue mixing while cooling to 45°C. Add perfume. Stir to 30°C.

To reduce oiliness, replace 5% of mineral oil with ACETULAN and an additional 10% of the mineral oil with isopropyl myristate. For satiny feel, replace part of Beeswax with PPG-36 Oleate. For dry film feel, add 2-5% GLUCAM P-20 to water phase.

#10
(Heavy Duty, W/O)

Oil Phase

AMERCHOL® L-500	2.0
AMERCHOL® C	5.0
Microcrystalline wax, 170-175°F m.p.	10.0
Mineral oil, 180 vis.	29.0
Sorbitan sesquioleate	2.0

Water Phase

Water	50.0
Sorbitol solution, 70%	2.0
Perfume and Preservative	q.s.

Add the water phase at 85°C to the oil phase at 85°C while mixing.Continue mixing and cool to 50°C. Add perfume and stir to 40°C. Homogenize.

To reduce oiliness, replace part to mineral oil with ACETULAN. To reduce tackiness, replace sorbitol with GLUCAM P-10. To impart slip, replace part of microcrystalline wax with cetyl alcohol.

#11
(Anti-Bacterial)

MACKANATE LO-SPECIAL	83.0
MACKAMIDE PKM	4.0
MACKERNIUM 007	0.8
Chloroxylenol	0.5
MACKSTAT DM	q.s.
Water, Fragrance qs to	100.0

Add MACKAMIDE PKM to MACKANATE LO-SPECIAL and heat to 70 degrees C. Blend until homogenous. Dissolve MACKERNIUM 007 in water and add to product. Blend until completely homogenous. Add Chloroxylenol. Cool to 50 degrees C. with mild agitation. Add MACKSTAT DM and fragrance and cool with continous agitation.

The product has cream pearlessent consistancy and can be packaged into a tube, jar or a high viscosity dispenser.

Vanishing Cream

#1

Phase 1

ROSSWAX 63-0412	8.0
ROSSWAX 573	12.0
AMERLATE P	1.0

EMEREST 2314	1.0
EMEREST 2316	1.0
Glyceryl Monostearate SE	.5

Phase 2

Water	99.0
EMERY 916 PURE GLYCERINE	8.0
Triethanolamine	1.2
Fragrance	q.s.
Preservative	q.s.

In separate steam jacketed kettles heat both phase 1 and 2 to temperature of 170F with agitation. When the temperature is reached add phase 1 to 2 with continued agitation cooling to 120 F to package. Fragrance may be added to the product as it is cooling.

#2
(Cleansing)

Oil Phase

SOLULAN® pb-10	8.2
ACETULAN®	2.0
Stearate acid, xxx	22.8
Isopropyl palmitate	5.0

Water Phase

Glycerine	4.0
Triethanolamine	1.2
Water	56.8
Perfume and Preservative	q.s.

Add the water phase at 85°C to the oil phase at 85°C while mixing. Continue mixing while cooling to 45°C. Add perfume, stir to 30°C.

To improve lubricity, replace isopropyl palmitate with AMERLATE P. To reduce tackiness, replace glycerine with GLUCAM P-10.

#3

(Pearlescent)

Oil Phase

AMERCHOL® 400	2.0
SOLULAN® PB-10	3.0
Stearic acid, xxx	20.0
Isopropyl palmitate	12.0

Water Phase

Glycerine	4.0
Triethanolamine	1.2
Water	57.8
Perfume and Preservative	q.s.

Add the water phase at 85°C to the oil phase at 85°C while mixing. Cool while mixing to 45°C. Add the perfume oil. Continue mixing while cooling to 30°C.

For complete rub-in, replace glycerine with GLUCAM E-20. To improve lubricity, replace part of isopropyl palmitate with AMERLATE P.

#4

(Almond with Collagen)

Phase 1

ROSSWAX 63-0412	5.90
ROSSWAX 573	8.90
AMERLATE P	.70
EMEREST 2314	.70
EMEREST 2316	.70
Glyceryl Monostearate SE	.37
ALMOND OIL-LIPOVOL ALM	1.00

Phase 2

EMERY 916 PURE GLYCERINE	6.00
Water	73.46
Triethanolamine	.90

Phase 3

COLLASOL	.37

Phase 4

GERMABEN II	1.00

In separate steam jacketed kettles heat both Phase (1) and (2) to a temperature of 170.F with agitation. When the temperature is reached, add Phase (1) to Phase (2) with continued agitation. Next add Phase (3) and then Phase (4) both with agitation, cool to 120.F and package.

#5
(Soft & Silky)

Part (A)

ROSSWAX 63-0412	8.0
ROSSWAX 573	10.0
ROSS LOTION OIL 2745	8.0
G M S-SE	.5

Part (B)

Water	97.0
Propylene glycol	8.0
Triethanolamine	2.0
GERMABEN II	1.2

Part (C)

Fragrance	q.s.

Heat Part (A) and Part (B) to 170.F in separate steam jacketed kettles under agitation. When fully heated add part (A) to Part (B) under agitation. Cool to 130.F. Add fragrance and package.

#6
(Apricot)

Phase (1)

ROSSWAX 63-0412	6.64
ROSSWAX 573	9.20
AMERLATE P	.80
EMEREST 2314	.80
EMEREST 2316	.80
Glyceryl Monostearate SE	.40
LIPOVOL P	1.30

Phase (2)

Water	71.9
EMERY 916 PURE GLYCERINE	6.20
Triethanolamine	.96

Phase (3)

GERMABEN II	1.0
FRAGRANCE GK-19	q.s.

In separate steam jacketed kettles, heat both Phase (1) and (2) to a temperature of 170.F with agitation. When the temperature is reached, add Phase (1) to Phase (2) with continued agitation. Cool to 130 F, add Phase (3) and fragrance. Continue to cool to 120 F and package.

Night Cream
#1

Oil Phase:

AMERCHOL® L-500	1.0
MODULAN®	2.0
Cocoa butter	7.0
SPERMWAX	4.0
Stearic acid, xxx	5.0

Cetyl alcohol	2.0
Silicone fluid 200, 350 cstks.	1.0
Glyceryl monostearate, neut.	5.0
Mineral oil 70 vis.	10.0

Water Phase:

Triethanlamine	1.5
Propylene glycol	4.0
Water	57.5
Perfume and Preservative	q.s.

Add the water phase at 85°C to the oil phase at 85°C while mixing. Continue mixing while cooling to 45°C, add perfume, mix to 30°C.

To reduce oily character, replace part of mineral oil with ACETULAN. For lighter residual feel, replace propylene glycol with GLUCAM E-10. For creamy elegance, replace part of stearic acid with AMERLATE LFA.

#2

Oil Phase:

AMERLATE® LFA	3.0
AMERLATE® P	1.5
AMERCHOL® C	4.0
Mineral oil, 70 vis.	3.5
Glyceryl monostearate, s.e.	6.0
Cetyl alcohol	3.0
Beeswax, USP	2.5
Spermwax	2.5

Water Phase:

Triethanolamine	1.0
Propylene glycol	2.5
Water	70.5
Perfume and Preservative	q.s.

Add water phase to oil phase at 80°C with good stirring. Cool while stirring to 45°C, add perfume, stir to 40°C.

To reduce tackiness, replace propylene glycol with GLUCAM E-10. To increase firmness, replace part of cetyl alcohol with stearyl alcohol.

#3
(Moisturizing)

Phase A	
Mineral Oil	10.00
CERAPHYL 368	2.00
EMERSOL 132	4.00
CERASYNT Q	3.00
MYRJ 52S	1.00
ABIL B8852	1.00
Lanolin Oil	0.50
Phase B	
Water	74.75
Triethanolamine: 99%	1.30
DERMACRYL 79	1.00
Phase C	
CARBOPOL 934	0.25
Phase D	
GERMABEN II-E	1.00
Phase E	
Fragrance	0.20

Heat water and triethanolamine to 80°C. Slowly sift in Dermacryl-79 and mix until completely dissolved. Slowly sift in Carbopol 934. In separate vessel, combine phase A and heat to 80°C until clear with mixing. Add Phase A to Phase B and mix thoroughly at 80°C for 30 minutes. Cool to 40°C, add Phase D and Phase E.

#4
(Moisterizing)

Oil Phase:	
OHlan™	0.5
Mineral oil, 80-90 vis.	11.0
Stearic acid, xxx	5.0

SPERMWAX	4.0
Glyceryl monostearate, s.e.	8.0
Water Phase:	
Triethanolamine	1.5
Propylene glycol	3.0
Water	67.0
Perfume and Preservative	q.s.

Add the water phase at 85°C to the oil phase at 85°C while mixing.Continue mixing while cooling to 45°C. Add perfume, stir to 30°C.

For improved texture, replace half the stearic acid with AMERLATE LFA. For reduced oiliness, replace paert of mineral oil with ACETULAN. For reduced tackiness, replace propylene glycol with GLUCAM E-10.

#5

(Glossy)

Oil Phase:	
AMERCHOL® C	4.0
AMERLATE® P	1.5
Stearic acid, xxx	3.0
Mineral oil, 70 vis.	3.5
Glyceryl monostearate, s.e.	6.0
Cetyl alcohol	3.0
Beeswax USP	2.5
Water Phase:	
Triethanolamine	1.0
Propylene glycol	2.5
Water	73.0
Perfume and Preservative	q.s.

Add water phase to oil phase at 85°C with good stirring. Cool and stir to 50°C. Add perfume and stir to 37°C.

For satiny feel, replace beeswax with PPG-36 Oleate. For reduced tackiness, replace propylene glycol with GLUCAM E-10. For reduced viscosity, replace part of cetyl alcohol with myristyl alcohol. For improved texture, replace stearic acid with AMERLATE LFA.

Skin Care Cream

I	APIFIL ®	8.00
	Cetyl Alcohol	1.00
	M.O.D. WL 2949	10.00
	ISOSTEARATE D'ISOSTEARYLE	7.00
	Wheat Germ Oil	3.00
	SILICONE 200 (100 CS)	1.00
	VEGETOL ® HUILEUX CALENDULA WL 1072	5.00
	Antioxygen	q.s.
II	DEMINERALIZED WATER	57.75
	CARBOPOL ® 934	0.30
	E.D.T.A.	0.05
	Triethanolamine 99% (50% solution)	0.60
	CEVENYL ®	1.00
	NUCLEODERM ® (2% aqueous solution)	5.00
	Preservative	q.s.
	Perfume	0.30

Disperse the CARBOPOL®. Let stand. Under moderate stirring, pour II heated up to 75°C into I heated up to 75°C. Then add the T.E.A. solution and the CEVENYL ® , cool down to 30°C while stirring. Add the other components.

Silk Protein Skin Cream

1.	Mineral Oil	10.0
2.	Coco Butter	2.0
3.	Cetearyl Alcohol & Ceteareth 20	4.0
4.	Emulsifying wax N.F.	6.0
5.	Stearic Acid	1.0
6.	Glyceryl Monostearate	2.8
7.	Glycerin	2.0
8.	Propylene Glycol	2.0
9.	Acetamide MEA 100%	0.5
10.	Triethanolamine	0.2
11.	MACKPRO NSP	1.5
12.	MACKSTAT DM	q.s.

13.	Fragrance	q.s.
14.	Deionized Water	q.s.

Melt 1,2,3,4,5,6,7,8,9, in a separate container to 75 degrees C. In the mixing tank heat the water to 78 degrees C. add 10, 11. Start mixing and add hot mixture of 1 thru 9 slowly with good agitation, mix for 20 minutes then start cooling. While mixing add at 50 degrees C. items 12 then 13 and mix until everything is homogeneous. Check pH and adjust if needed with triethanolamine or acid solution to 5.4 - 6.5.

Emollient Cream O/W

Oil Phase

GLUCATE® DO	1.5
GLUCAMATE® SSE-20	3.0
Petrolatum	8.0
Isopropyl Palmitate	3.0
Mineral Oil	6.0
Stearyl Alcohol	2.0
Cetyl Alcohol	1.0
Dimethicone	0.5

Water Phase

Magnesium Aluminum silicate (4% aqueous dispersion)	25.0
Xanthan Gum	0.3
Water	49.7
Perfume & Preservatives	q.s.

Disperse the xanthan gum in water with vigorous agitation while heating to 70°C. Heat the magnesium aluminum silicate dispersion to 70°C with vigorous agitation. Heat oil phase to 70°C. Add the two aqueous dispersions, one at a time, to the oil phase with vigorous agitation. Continue agitating while cooling to room temperature. Add perfume below 40°C.

Daily Skin Care Cream

Oil Phase

GLUCAM E-20 Distearate	2.5
GLUCATE DO	2.0
GLUCATE SS	2.5
PROPAL	3.0

Water Phase

Deionized water	77.0
Carbomer 934 (3% aq.)	10.0
Triethanolamine (10% aq.)	3.0
Perfume and preservative	q.s.

Heat oil phase to 80°C. Heat water phase minus the triethanolamine to 80°C. Add water phase to oil phase at 80°C. Immediately add the triethanolamine. Cool to 40°C while mixing. Add perfume at 40°C and continue to cool to room temperature and pack.

Dry Skin Cream
#1

Phase A

QUATRISOFT™POLYMER LM-200	0.2
Water	36.1

Phase B

Carbomer 940	0.2
Water	39.8
Triethanolamine (99%)	0.2

Phase C

Propylene Glycol	3.0
GLUCAMATE® SSE-20	3.5

Phase D

AMERCHOL-L101®	8.0
MODULAN®	1.0
Glyceryl Monostearate, Neutral	2.0
GLUCATE® SS	1.5
Mineral Oil	4.5
Perfume and Preservative	q.s.

Disperse QUATRISOFT™ POLYMER LM-200 in water at room temperature with good agitation. When thoroughly dispersed, heat to 75°C until uniform. Mix phase B separately until uniform at room temperature. Add phase A to phase B, minus triethanolamine with mixing. When thoroughly mixed, add the triethanolamine with mixing until gel-like. Heat AB and phase C to 75°C. Add phase C to AB. Heat phase D to 75°C and add to ABC. Cool to room temperature with mixing.

#2

Part (A)	
MODULAN	3.7
AMERCHOL L-101	4.2
Isopropyl Myristate	2.7
Sodium Stearate Pure	10.0
Glyceryl Mono Stearate Se	1.8
ROSS SPERMACETTI WAX SUB. 573	5.5
ROSS JOJOBA OIL	1.8
Part (B)	
Water	59.7
EMERY 916 GLYCERINE PURE	9.2
Triethanolamine	1.4
Part (C)	
Preservative	q.s.
Part (D)	
Fragrance	q.s.

Melt Part (A) and Part (B) in separate vessels to 170.F under agitation. When temperature is reached, mix Part (A) to Part (B) and cool. Package in containers at below 120.F.

#3
(O/W)

Oil Phase:	
PROMULGEN® D	0.7
GLUCAM ® P-20 DISTEARATE	2.0
GLUCATE® DO	0.5
ACETULAN®	2.0
CETAL	1.0
Stearic Acid, xxx	4.0
Mineral Oil, 70 vis.	5.0
Cetyl Palmitate	1.0
Water Phase:	
Carbomer 934	0.3
Triethanolamine (10% aqueous)	17.0

Water	66.5
Perfume and Preservative	q.s.

Disperse the carbomer 934 in water with vigorous agitation. Heat the oil and water phases, minus the triethanolamine, to 85°C. Add water phase to oil phase with moderate agitation. Immediately add the triethanolamine. Mix while cooling to room temperature. Add perfume at 40°C.

#4
(W/O)

Oil Phase:

GLUCATE® DO	3.0
AMERCHOL® L-500	3.5
Talc	5.0
Ceresin	4.0
PROMYR	5.0
Aluminum Stearate	2.0
Mineral Oil, 70 vis.	12.5

Water Phase:

Water	65.0
Perfume & Preservative	q.s.

Combine the oil phase ingredients and mix while heating to 90°C to disperse the aluminum stearate. Heat the water to 75°C while cooling the oil phase to 75°C with continued agitation. At 75°C, add the water to the oil phase with good mixing. Continue agitating while cooling to room temeperature. Add perfume below 40°C. Homogenize and pack.

#5
(All-Purpose)

Water Phase:

GLUCQUAT 100	1.0
Deionized water	83.0

Oil Phase:

GLUCAM P-20 DISTEARATE	2.0
GLUCATE DO	0.5

PROMULGEN D	4.5
ACETULAN	2.0
CETAL	1.0
Mineral oil, 70 vis.	5.0
Cetyl Palmitate	1.0
Perfume and preservative	q.s.

Dissolve GLUQUAT 100 into deionized water, and heat to 80°C with adequate agitation. Combine oil phase ingredients, and heat to 80°C with propeller mixing. Slowly add water phase to oil phase, and mix until uniform. When material starts to thicken during cooling, change to slow sweep agitation.

#6

(W/O)

I	APIFAC®	12.00
	Mineral Oil	10.00
	M.O.D. WL 2949	6.00
II	Demineralized Water	63.30
	CARBOPOL ® 934	0.30
	Glycerin	5.00
	Preservative	q.s.
	Triethanolamine 99% (50% solution)	0.60
	CEVENYL ®	2.00
	Racemic Alphabisabolol	0.50
	Perfume	0.30

Disperse the CARBOPOL ®. Let stand. Pour II heated up to 80°C into I heated up to 80°C. Add the T.E.A. solution and the CEVENYL ® and stir quickly. Then cool down with normal stirring. Around 30-35°C, add the other components.

Moisturizing Cream

#1

A	VEEGUM® PRO	1.5
	Water	74.5
B	Triethanolamine	1.0
	Glycerin	4.0

C	Stearate Acid XXX	2.0
	Cetyl alcohol	2.0
	Isopropyl myristate	2.0
	ATMUL 124	3.0
	MARCOL 130	10.0
	Preservative	q.s.

Heat the water to 70 to 75°C, then slowly add the VEEGUM PRO while agitating at maximum available shear. Mix until smooth. Add B to A with slow mixing until smooth. Maintain A/B at 70 to 75°C; heat C to 70 to 75°C. Add C to A/B and mix until cool.

Consistency; Medium viscosity cream.

Suggested Packaging; Wide mouth jar.

#2

Phase A:	
Water	57.40
Glycerin	3.00
CARBOPOL 940	0.70
Disodium EDTA	0.10
Methylparaben	0.25
Phase B:	
PEG-8	5.00
HETESTER PCA	8.00
MYRJ 52S	0.50
Cetyl Alcohol	1.00
Propylparaben	0.10
EUTANOL G	4.00
Stearyl Alcohol	1.00
CETIOL LC	3.00
CARNATION MINERAL OIL	8.00
CERASYNT Q	3.00
Perfluorpolymethylisopropylether	2.00

Phase C	
Triethanolamine, 99%	0.70
Phase D	
Water	2.00
GERMALL 115	0.25

Heat Phase A to 80°C. Heat Phase B to 80°C. Add Phase B to Phase A. Cool to 75°C and add Phase C. Continue cooling to 30°C and add Phase D.

#3

Part A	
POLAWAX	10.00
INCROQUAT BEHENYL TMS	3.00
Mineral Oil	5.00
Part B	
Deionized Water	80.00
Part C	
HYDROLACTIN 2500	1.00
GERMABEN II	1.00

Combine ingredients of Part A with mixing and heat to 70°C. Heat Part B to 70°C. Add Part B to Part A with good mixing. Continue mixing and cool to 45°C. Add Part C with mixing and cool to desired fill temperature.

Properties:
pH= 4.8
Brookfield Viscosity RV#6 @ 50rpm=10.400cps

#4
(Deep)

Part A	
POLAWAX	2.00
SYNCROWAX AW1-C	5.50
SYNCROWAX HGL-C	1.00
CRODALAN LA	1.00

SUPER REFINED™ COCONUT OIL	3.00
SUPER HARTOLAN	1.00
CRODAMOL PMP	7.00
Petrolatum	1.00
Propyl Paraben	.20

Part B

Water, deionized	66.00
Methyl paraben	.30
Glycerin	10.00
Triethanolamine (99%)	1.00

Part C

CROMOIST CS	1.00

Combine the ingredients of Part A with mixing and heat to 75°C. Combine the ingredients of Part B with mixing and heat to 75°C. Add Part B to Part A with homogenizer mixing and cool to 65°C. Continue mixing with a sweep blade mixer and cool to 40°C. Add Part C with mixing and cool to desired fill temperature.

#5
(Replenishing)

Part I

Water	81.6
MONAQUAT P-TS	3.0

Part II

Cetyl Alcohol (95%)	5.0
Myristyl Myristate	5.0
Isopropyl Myristate	4.0
Lanolin Alcohol	0.4
Dimethicone (350 C.S.)	1.0

Heat Part I to 65°C. Mix until uniform. Heat Part II to 65°C. Mix until uniform. Add Part II to Part I with stirring. Cool slowly to 40°C and add fragrance, coloring, or preservative as required. Cool with stirring to 35°C, fill.

Therapeutic Humectant Creme

Part I	
Deionized Water	66.8
MONAQUAT P-TS	3.0
Glycerin (99%)	15.0
Part II	
Cetyl alcohol (95%)	5.0
Myristyl Myristate	5.0
C_{12}-C_{15} Alcohols Benzoate	3.0
Propylene Glycol Monostearate (Pure)	2.2

Heat Part I to 65°C, with mixing, until clear. Heat Part II to 65°C, with mixing. Slowly add Part II to Part I with efficient mixing. Remove heat after 5 mintues. Cool slowly. Product will start to thicken at about 50°C. If propeller slows down, increase speed to ensure efficient mixing. Add fragrance, coloring or preservative as required. Cool to 40°C, fill.

Cold Cream with Jojoba Oil

Part A	1.	2.	3.
ROSS BEESWAX SUBSTITUTE 628/5	11.0	13.0	13.0
ROSS FULLY REFINED PARAFIN WAX 150/160	2.0	0.0	0.0
Mineral Oil 80/90	45.5	47.5	45.5
Glycerol Monostearate S.E.	0.3	0.3	0.3
ROSS JOJOBA OIL	2.0	0.0	2.0
Part B			
Borax	0.8	.8	.8
Water	38.4	38.4	38.4
Fragrance	q.s	q.s	q.s
Preservative	q.s	q.s	q.s

Heat Part A to 170.F and agitate. Heat Part B to 170.F and agitate. Cool to 160.F and add Part A to Part B at 160.F with good agitation. Cool slowly with agitation and pour at 110.F.

European Performing Cream

The combination of ingredients in this formula produce an elegant cream which moisturizes and promotes healthy skin. The SUPER REFINED OILS used were selected to impart a light emollient feel to skin. CRODAMOL PTIS and CRODAMOL PMP modify the formula to provide a powdery feel.

Part A	
Deionized Water	69.5
Carbomer 940	0.2
Glycerin	2.0
TEA (99%)	0.4
Part B	
Mineral Oil	1.5
SUPER REFINED ™ OLIVE OIL	1.0
CRODAMOL PMP	5.0
FLUILAN	2.0
POLAWAX	4.0
SQUALENE	1.5
CRODAMOL PTIS	2.0
VOLPO 5	1.0
VOLPO 10	2.0
CHOLESTEROL NF	0.5
SUPER REFINED ™ GRAPESEED OIL	0.2
NOVOL	0.6
Dimethicone D/C 200 200cps	0.5
Part C	
Vitamin E (Liquid)	0.1
GERMABEN II	1.0
Part D	
Deionized Water	4.8
Allantoin	0.2

Combine the water and glycerine of Part A with mixing. Dust in the Carbomer 940 with good mixing and allow to hydrate. Heat with mixing. to 70°C, and add the TEA. Combine ingredients of Part B with mixing and heat to 70°C. Add Part B to Part A with good mixing and cool to 45°C. Add Part

C ingredients individually with mixing. Combine Part D ingredients with mixing and mix until uniform. Add Part D with mixing and cool to desired fill temperature.

Properties:
pH 7.45
Viscosity RV7 @ 50rpm=8,800cps

Skin Conditioning Cream

Water Phase	
KYTAMER™ PC	0.5
GLUCAM® E-10	5.0
GLUCAMATE® SSE-20	1.0
Deionized Water	65.5
Oil Phase	
PROMULGEN® G	5.0
AMERCHOL L-101	4.0
AMERLATE® P	3.0
GLUCATE® SS	1.0
Mineral Oil	15.0
Perfume and Preservative	q.s.

Disperse KYTAMER™ PC in water with high speed agitation. When completely dispersed heat to 75°C with continuous mixing until clear and uniform. Add GLUCAMATE® SSE-20 while maintaining temperature of water phase at 75°C. Heat oil phase to 75°C. Add water phase at 75°C to oil phase at 75°C with good agitation. Continue mixing while slowly cooling to room temperature. Add perfume below 50°C.

Hands, Face and Body Nourisher, W/O

A	VEEGUM	1.25
	Water	49.60
	Sodium borate	0.15

B	Sorbitol 70%	21.60
	ARLACEL 186	2.40
	MARCOL 130	14.50
	Petrolatum	5.00
	NIMLESTEROL D	2.50
	WAXENOL 821 S.B.	3.00
	Preservative	q.s.

Slowly add VEEGUM to the water, while agitating at maximum available shear. Continue mixing until smooth. Slowly add sodium borate, mixing until uniform. Heat A to 75°C. Heat B to 75°C. Add A to B and mix until smooth and uniform.

Consistency: Medium viscosity cream.
Suggested Packaging: Jar or squeeze tube.

Ultra Rich Hand and Body Nourisher

VEEGUM Ultra thickens and stabilizes this creamy, oil-in-water emulsion prepared using a non-ionic emulsifier system. It features the "dry touch" application properties typical of formulas containing VEEGUM. LIPACIDE PCO functions as an anti-irritant that complements the group of oil phase emollients. VEEGUM *Ultra* whitens and brightens this cosmetic formula and adjusts the pH to approximate that of normal skin.

A	VEEGUM® *Ultra*	1.50
	Deionized Water	79.00
B	Glycerin	3.00
	Aloe Vera Gel	2.00
C	LIPACIDE® PCO	1.00
	Cetyl Esters	1.00
	Glyceryl Stearate SE	2.50
	Isopropyl Palmitate	5.00
	Sorbitan Palmitate	2.25
	Polysorbate 40	2.75

D	Preservative, Fragrance	q.s.

Heat the water to 55°C. Add VEEGUM *Ultra* slowly while mixing at 500 rpm with a propeller stirrer. Increase mixer to 1500-1700rpm and mix for 30 minutes while maintaining temperature at 55°C. Add B to A and mix until uniform. Heat C to 60°C and add to (A and B). Mix (A, B and C) for 30 minutes. Avoid air entrapment. Slow mixer to 1000 rpm and mix while cooling to 35°C. Add D and mix until uniform. Package.

Properties:

Viscosity	2200 cps
pH	5.3
Color	Bright,White

Hand Cream

#1

I	EMULCIRE ® 61 WL 2659	10.00
	Stearic Acid	2.00
	M.O.D. WL 2949	5.00
	SILICONE 100 (100CS)	0.50
II	Demineralized Water	79.30
	Glycerin	3.00
	Preservative	q.s.
	Perfume	0.20

Under stirring pour II heated up to 75°C into I heated up to 75°C. Cool while stirring and around 30°C, add the other components.

#2

(Soft)

Oil Phase

AMERCHOL L-101®	5.0
MODULAN®	5.0
SOLULAN® 16	1.0
Petrolatum, USP white	5.0

Water Phase

CARBOPOL 934	0.75
Water	77.25
Sodium hydroxide, 10% aq.	2.25
ETHOMEEN C-25, 10% aq.	3.75
Perfume and Preservative	q.s.

Disperse the Carbopol in the water with high speed agitation. Mix until free from lumps. Heat to 70°C. Add sodium hydroxide and Ethomeen C-25 solutions. Add oil phase at 70°C with good stirring. Stir to 45°C. Add perfume, continue stirring to 30°C.

To reduce tackiness, add 2% GLUCAM P-10 to water phase. For added emollience and emulsion stabilization, replace petrolatum with AMERCHOL CAB.

#3

(Firm)

Oil Phase

AMERCHOL L-101®	4.0
ACETULAN®	2.0
Isopropyl palmitate	2.0
Stearic acid, xxx	2.0
Cetyl alcohol	0.5
Stearyl alcohol	0.5
ARLACEL 165	5.0
Silicone fluid 200, 350 cstks.	1.0

Water Phase

ALBAGEL	1.5
Propylene glycol	5.0
Water	76.5
Perfume and Preservative	q.s.

Disperse the Albagel in the water at 80°C using high speed mixing. Add the water phase at 80°C to the oil phase at 80°C while mixing. Continue mixing and cool to 50°C. Add perfume. Stir to 35°C.

To reduce tackiness, replace propylene glycol with GLUCAM E-10. To impart satiny feel, replace silicone fluid with PPG-36 Oleate. For softer texture, replace stearyl alcohol with myristyl alcohol and replace stearic acid with AMERLATE LFA.

#4
(Protective)

Oil Phase	
AMERCHOL® CAB	5.0
AMERLATE® LFA	3.5
PROMULGEN® D	2.0
Glyceryl Stearate	5.0
Dimethicone	20.0
Water Phase	
Water	64.0
Triethanolamine	0.5
Perfume and Preservative	q.s.

Heat both phases to 75°C. Add water phase to oil phase at 75°C and mix while cooling. Pour at 35°C.

Lotions

#1
(Nonionic All-Purpose O/W)

Water Phase	
POLYOX WSR N-12K	0.10
GLUCAM E-20	5.00
Deionized water	75.90
Oil Phase	
GLUCATE SS	1.00
GLUCAMATE SSE-20	3.00
ACETULAN	2.00
CETAL	2.00
Glyceryl Monostearate (neutral)	1.00
Sesame Oil	10.00
Perfume and Preservative	q.s.

Add POLYOX WSR N-12K to GLUCAM E-20 and mix to form a slurry. Add slurry to room temperature water until uniform. Heat to 80°C. Separately heat oil phase to 80°C. Add water phase to oil phase at 80°C. Cool while mixing to room temperature.

#2

(All Skin Type)

Oil Phase	
AMERCHOL® L-500	0.80
SOLULAN® PB-20	7.50
SOLULAN® C-24	0.30
Isopropyl palmitate	10.00
Stearic acid, xxx	2.00
Glyceryl monostearate, neut.	1.00
Water Phase	
Water	77.28
CARBOPOL 941	0.12
Triethanolamine	1.00
Perfume and Preservative	q.s.

Disperse Carbopol thoroughly in water while stirring at 85°C. Add triethanolamine. Add water phase to oil phase at 85°C with good stirring. Cool with stirring to 45°C. Add perfume, continue stirring to 30°C.

To impart satiny-feel, with heavier body, replace 1-2 parts of isopropyl palmitate with PPG-36 oleate. To impart slip, replace 1-2 parts of isopropyl palmitate with cetyl alcohol. These additions will also increase viscosity.

#3

(All Skin Types)

Oil Phase	
AMERCHOL L-101®	5.0
SOLULAN® 98	2.0
Cetyl alcohol	1.0
MONAMID 718	1.0
ARLACEL 165	4.0

Water Phase

Water	87.0
Citric acid solution, 20% in water q.s. to pH 5.5	
Perfume and Preservative	q.s.

Heat water and oil phases to 85°C. Add water phase to oil phase with good stirring. Continue stirring while cooling to 45°C. Add perfume oil and citric acid solution. Stir to 30°C.

To increase viscosity, replace part of cetyl alcohol with stearyl alcohol. To decrease viscosity, replace part of cetyl alcohol with myristyl alcohol. To provide humectancy add GLUCAM E-20 to water phase.

#4
(Moisturizing)

Oil Phase

AMERLATE® P	0.5
Stearic acid, xxx	3.0
Glyceryl monostearate, neut.	2.0

Water Phase

GLUCAM® E-10	15.0
Triethanolamine	1.0
Water	78.5
Perfume and Preservative	q.s.

Heat both phases to 85°C. Add water to oil with good stirring. Cool while stirring to 45°C. Add perfume, stir to 30°.
Consistency and lubricity can be increased by raising concentration of AMERLATE P.

#5
(Mild)

Oil Phase

GLUCATE SS	0.5
GLUCAMATE SSE-20	1.5
CETAL	0.5

Mineral Oil, 70 vis.	5.0
Squalane	0.9

Water Phase

Water	73.8
Carbomer 934 (3% aq.)	10.0
Triethanolamine (10% aq.)	3.0
BIOCARE POLYMER HA-24	3.8
GERMABEN IIE	1.0

Heat oil and water phases to 75°C and combine with good agitation. Add triethanolamine and Germaben IIE. BioCare Polymer HA-24 is added at 35-40°C with thorough agitation.

#6

(All-Purpose Conditioning)

Oil Phase

PROMULGEN G	5.0
GLUCATE SS	2.0
GLUCAMATE SSE-20	2.0
SOLULAN 5	0.5
Mineral Oil, 70 vis.	2.0

Water Phase

BIOCARE POLYMER HA-24	3.8
GLUCAM E-10	3.5
Water	80.2
GERMABEN IIE	1.0

Add water phase (minus the BioCare Polymer HA-24 and Germaben IIE) at 85°C to the oil phase at 85°C with mixing. Add the Germaben IIE at 75°C. Continue to mix to 40°C. Add the BioCare Polymer HA-24 with mixing while cooling to 30°C.

#7

(Mild Luxurious Cationic)

Part A

INCROQUAT BEHENYL TMS	3.5
POLAWAX	3.0
CRODACOL S-95	1.0

CRODAMOL PMP	3.0
CRODAMOL PTC	2.0
CARNATION MINERAL OIL	3.0
SNOW WHITE PETROLATUM	2.0
Dimethicone 350cs (200fl)	0.5

Part B

Water, deionized	73.0
Glycerin	8.0

Part C

GERMABEN II	1.0

Combine ingredients of Part A with mixing and heat to 75°C. Combine ingredients of Part B with mixing and heat to 75°C. Add Part B to Part A with good mixing. Continue mixing and cool to 45°C. Add Part C with mixing and cool to desired fill temperature.

#8
(High Petrolatum)

Part A

PERLATUM 410	30.00
CRODAMOL PMP	10.00
VOLPO 3	2.30

Part B

Deionized Water	45.35
CARBOPOL 941	0.13
10% Sodium Hydroxide Solution	0.52

Part C

Glycerine	5.00
VOLPO S-10	5.70

Part D

GERMABEN II	1.00

Dust the Carbomer 941 of Part B into the water with mixing. Heat to 80°C and add the Sodium Hydroxide Solution. Combine ingredients of Part C with mixing and heat to 80°C. Add Part C to Part B with mixing. Combine ingredients of Part A with mixing and heat to 80°C. Add combined Parts B and C to Part A with mixing and cool to 40°C. Add Part D with mixing and cool to desired fill temperature.

#9

(Low solids Almond)

Water	568
Carbomer 934	2
ROSSWAX 573	4
GMS SE	4
LIPOVAL AIM	16
Coconut Oil	16
Jojoba Oil	4
TEA	4
GERMABEN II	6
Fragrance GG-44	q.s.

Heat the water to 60.C under agitation and slowly add the Carbomer 934. When the water is fully mixed add the 573, GMS, Almond Oil, Coconut Oil, and Jojoba Oil that have been heated to 65.C in a separate kettle. As soon as they have been mixed well add the preservative, the fragrance and then the TEA under high agitation. Cool the batch to 55.C. and package.

#10

(Low Cost Low Solids)

Water	500
Carbomer 934	4
ROSSWAX 573	4
GMS SE	4
Jojoba Oil	3
DOW CORNING SILICONE 344	6
Triethanolamine	4
Perfume	q.s.
GERMABEN II	q.s.

Heat the water under agitation and slowly add the Carbomer 934. When fully mixed add the 573, GMS, Jojoba Oil and Silicone that have been blended in a separate kettle maintaining a temperature of 140.F. As soon as all the ingredients have been mixed well add the Preservatives, the Perfume, and add the TEA, under high agitation, cool to 120.F. and package.

#11
(Soft & Silky)

Part A	
ROSSWAX 63-0412	1.6
ROSSWAX 1641	1.2
ROSSWAX 63-0212	1.0
G M S-SE	2.1
ROSS LOTION OIL 2745	9.4
Part B	
Water	78.0
Propylene Glycol	4.7
GERMABEN II	1.0
Triethanolamine	1.0
Part C	
Fragrance	q.s.

Heat Part (A) and Part (B) to 170.F in separate steam jacket kettles under agitation. When fully heated, add Part (A) to Part (B) under agitation. Cool to 130.F, Fragrance and package.

#12
(O/W)

Phase 1	
ROSS WAX 63-0412	1.6
ROSS WAX 1641	1.0
MINERAL OIL #9	2.1
ROSS WAX 63-0212	1.0
AMERCHOL L-101	5.2
ROSS JOJOBA OIL	2.1
GMS SE	2.1

Phase 2

Triethanolamine	1.0
Propylene glycol	4.7
Water	78.2
GERMABEN II	1.0
NOVAROME DE47 FRAGRANCE	q.s.

In separate kettles bring Phase (1) and (2) to 170.F. When temperature is reached add Phase (1) to (2) with agitation. Cool to 120.F and package.

#13
(Cleansing)

Oil Phase

AMERCHOL L-101®	3.0
ACETULAN®	2.0
Stearate acid, xxx	2.0
Glyceryl monostearate, neut.	2.5
SOLULAN® 16	2.0
Mineral oil, 70 vis.	15.0

Water Phase

Glycerine	4.0
Triethanolamine	0.4
Water	69.1
Perfume and Preservative	q.s.

Add water to oil phase at 85°C with good stirring. Cool while stirring to 45°C. Add perfume, cool while stirring to 30°C.

To reduce oily feel, replace part of the mineral oil with AMERLATE P and cetyl alcohol. To improve rinsability, replace half the mineral oil with diglycol laurate. To reduce tack, replace glycerine with GLUCAM P-20.

#14
(Cleansing)
(High Viscosity)

Oil Phase

GLUCATE® SS	1.2
AMERCHOL ® L-500	1.0
Beeswax	2.0

SPERMWAX	2.0
Mineral oil, 70 vis.	16.0

Water Phase

GLUCAMATE® SSE-20	2.0
CARBOPOL 941	0.2
Water	73.6
Triethanolamine (10% aqueous)	2.0
Perfume and Preservative	q.s.

Disperse the Carbopol in the water using high speed mixing. Mix until free from lumps. Add the GLUCAMATE SSE-20 and heat while mixing. Add the water phase at 85°C. to the oil phase at 85°C while mixing. After the emulsion has formed and the temperature drops to 60°C, add the triethanolamine. Stir and cool to 45°C. Add perfume, stir to 35°C.

To impart improved rinse-off properties to cleanser, replace part of mineral oil with diglycol laurate. To improve spreading characteristics, replace part of mineral oil with AMERLATE P. To reduce viscosity, replace beeswax with cetyl alcohol.

#15
(Silk Protein)

1.	Mineral Oil	3.00
2.	MACKESTER SP	2.00
3.	Emulsifying Wax N.F.	3.00
4.	Glyceryl Stearate & PEG-100 Stearate	2.00
5.	Polysorbate 80	0.66
6.	Sorbitan Palmitate	0.60
7.	Glycerin	2.00
8.	Acetamide MEA 100%	1.00
9.	MACKPRO NSP	2.50
10.	MACKSTAT DM	q.s.
11.	Fragrance	q.s.
12.	Deionized Water	q.s.

Melt 1,2,3,4,5,6,7,8, in a separate container to 75 degrees C. In the mixing tank heat the water #12 to 78 degrees C. and add #9. Start mixing and add the hot mixture of 1 thru 8 slowly with good agitation and mix well for 20 minutes. Then start slow cooling with good mixing without aeration. At 45 degrees C. add #10 and #11 and mix in. Check pH and adjust if needed to 4.8 - 5.8. Mix until cool.

#16

(Silk Protein)

1.	White Petrolatum	2.6
2.	MACKOL 1618	4.0
3.	Sorbitan Oleate	1.2
4.	Polysorbate 80	0.7
5.	MACKERNIUM SDC-85	1.5
6.	MACKAMIDE AME-75	0.5
7.	MACKPRO NSP	1.0
8.	Silicone Copolyol	0.1
9.	MACKSTAT DM	q.s.
10.	Fragrance	q.s.
11.	Deionized Water	q.s.

Melt 1,2,3,4,5,6, in a separate container to 75 degrees C. In the mixing tank heat the water #11 to 78 degrees C. Add #7 and #8. Start mixing and add hot mixture 1 thru 6 slowly with good agitation, mix for 20 minutes then start cooling while mixing. Mix well for 20 minutes then start slow cooling while mixing avoid aeration. At 45 degrees C. add 9 and 10 add mix, check pH 5 - 6 adjust if needed, mix until cool.

#17

(Dry skin)

Oil Phase	
AMERCHOL L-101®	8.0
MODULAN®	1.0
Stearic acid, xxx	2.5
Glyceryl monostearate, neut.	2.0
Mineral oil, 70 vis.	4.5
Water Phase	
Water	76.5
Propylene glycol	4.5
Triethanolamine	1.0
Perfume and Preservative	q.s.

Heat oil and water phases to 85°C. Add water to oil with good stirring. Cool while stirring to 45°C, add perfume. Stir to 30°C.

To reduce oily feeling, replace part of mineral oil with isopropyl myristate, or ACETULAN. Mineral oil can be increased up to 15% without upsetting emulsifier balance.

#18
(Dry Skin)

A	VEEGUM	1.40
	RHODIGEL 23	0.35
	Water	72.25
	Glycerin	4.00
B	ACETULAN	4.00
	FINSOLV TN	4.00
	POLYSYNLANE	3.00
	Cocoa butter	4.00
	Petrolatum	2.00
	ARLACEL 165	5.00
	Preservative	q.s.

Add the dry blend of VEEGUM and Rhodigel to the water slowly, agitating at maximum available shear until smooth. Add the glycerin and heat A to 65-70°C. Heat B to 65-70°C. Add B to A and mix while cooling. Pour off at about 40°C.

Consistency/Suggested Packaging: Medium viscosity lotion/plastic squeeze bottle.

#19
(Dry Skin)

Oil Phase

Propylene Glycol Monostearate	3.0
CETAL	1.0
Stearic Acid	2.5
PROMYR	1.0

Water Phase

GLUCAM® E-10	5.0
Triethanolamine	0.8
Water	86.7
Perfume and Preservative	q.s.

Heat the oil and water phases to 80°C. Add water phase to the oil phase with moderate agitation. Mix while cooling to room temperature. Add perfume below 40°C and pack.

#20

(Dry Skin)

Oil Phase

AMERCHOL L-101®	8.0
MODULAN®	1.0
AMERLATE® LFA	3.0
Glyceryl monostearate, neut.	5.0
Mineral oil, 70 vis.	4.5

Water Phase

Triethanolamine	1.0
Propylene glycol	4.5
Water	73.0
Perfume and Preservative	q.s.

Add the water phase at 85°C to the oil phase at 85°C while stirring. Stir and cool to 45°C. Add perfume, stir to 30°C.

For more complete rub-in, replace part of mineral oil with isopropyl palmitate and propylene glycol with GLUCAM E-10. For greater skin treatment increase MODULAN.

#21

(W/O)

Oil Phase

AMERCHOL L-101®	5.0
Petrolatum	5.0
Mineral oil, 70 vis.	33.5
Lanolin	3.0
Sorbitan sesquioleate	2.5

Beeswax	4.0
GLUCATE® SS	0.5
Water Phase	
VEEGUM REGULAR	0.5
Borax	0.5
GLUCAM® E-20	2.0
Water	43.5
Perfume and Preservative	q.s.

Disperse Veegum thoroughly in water at 85°C with high speed mixing. Add water to oil at 85°C with good stirring. Stir and cool to 45°C, add perfume. Stir and cool to 30°C.

To achieve more complete rub-in on skin, replace large part of mineral oil with AMERLATE P, ACETULAN and cetyl alcohol mixture.

#22

(Emollient Dry Touch)

A	VEEGUM	0.5
	Water	85.5
B	Triethanolamine	0.1
	Glycerin	3.5
C	CARNATION WHITE MINERAL OIL	3.6
	Petrolatum	0.4
	Stearic acid	1.6
	Cetyl alcohol	0.8
	KESSCO GLYCEROL MONOSTEARATE S.E.	1.4
	ACETULAN	2.0
	DOW CORNING 200 FLUID (350 cs)	0.6
	Preservative	q.s.

Slowly add VEEGUM to the water, while agitating at maximum available shear. Continue mixing until smooth. Add B to A and heat to 70-75°C with gentle stirring. Heat C to 75-80°C. Add C to A/B and mix thoroughly while cooling.

Consistency: Medium viscosity lotion.
Suggested Packaging: Squeeze or pump bottle.

#23
(Emollient)

A	VEEGUM® PRO	1.5
	Water	83.8
B	Triethanolamine	0.1
	Glycerin	3.5
C	MARCOL 130	3.6
	Petrolatum	0.4
	Stearic acid XXX	1.6
	Cetyl alcohol	1.5
	KESSCO GLYCEROL MONOSTEARATE SE	1.4
	ACETULAN	2.0
	DOW CORNING 200 FLUID	0.6
	Preservative	q.s.

Heat the water to 70 to 75°C, then slowly add the VEEGUM PRO while agitating at maximum available shear. Mix until smooth. Add B to A with slow agitation until smooth. Maintain A/B at 70 to 75°C, heat C to 75 to 80°C. Add C to A/B and mix until cool.

Consistency: Medium viscosity lotion.
Suggested Packaging: Squeeze or pump bottle.

#24
(Jojoba)

Part A

MODULAN®	1.6
AMERCHOL L-101	.8
Isopropl Palmitate	5.0
Glyceryl Mono Stearate Pure	2.1
ROSSWAX 63-0412	4.0
Isopropl Myristate	4.0
ROSS JOJOBA OIL	1.6

Part B

Water	74.4
EMERY 916	4.2
Triethanolamine	2.3

Heat Part (A) and Part (B) in separate vessels to 170.F under agitation. When temperature is reached mix Part (A) to Part (B), and cool. Package in container at below 120.F.

#25

(Silicone Barrier)

A	VEEGUM	1.00
	RHODIGEL 23	0.25
	Water	80.75
B	SILICONE 556 FLUID	5.00
	Stearic acid (triple pressed)	5.00
	TWEEN 20	4.50
	ARLACEL 20	3.50
	Preservative	q.s.

Add the VEEGUM/Rhodigel dry blend to the water slowly, agitating at maximum available shear until smooth. Heat A to 70°C. Heat B ingredients to 75°C. Add B to A and mix until cool.

Consistency/Suggested Packaging: lotion/plastic squeeze bottle

#26

(Facial)

Phase A:

PROMULGEN® D	1.5
Stearic Acid, xxx	3.0
AMERCHOL L-101®	5.0
ACETULAN®	2.0
Cetyl Palmitate	1.0
OHlan®	0.5

Phase B:

Carbomer 934 (3% aqueous)	10.0
Water	65.0

Phase C:	
Triethanolamine (10% aqueous)	12.0
Perfume and Preservative	q.s.

Heat all phases to 80°C. Begin mixing at 80°C phase B to phase A. Upon completion of phasing, immediately add phase C. Mix well while slowly cooling to 35°C, at which time perfume may be added. Mix and cool to room temperature.

#27

(Facial)

Oil Phase:	
PROMULGEN® D	4.5
AMERCHOL L-101®	5.0
OHLAN®	0.5
ACETULAN®	2.0
Cetyl Palmitate	1.0
Water Phase:	
Water	87.0
Perfume and Preservative	q.s.

Heat both phases to 80°C. Add water phase to oil phase at 80°C and continue to mix until 40°C. Add perfume at 40°C. continue to mix until room temperature.

#28

(Face, Extra Sensitive)

Part A	
CRODAMOL PMP	5.00
FLUILAN	2.00
CRODAMOL PTIS	5.00
ESCALOL® 507	7.00
UVINUL M-40	3.00
VOLPO-5	1.00
VOLPO 10	2.00
POLAWAX	4.00

Part B

Deionized Water	64.35
CARBOPOL 934	0.25
Triethanolamine (99%)	0.40
Glycerin	5.00

Part C

GERMABEN II	1.00

Dust in the Carbopol 934 of Part B into the water with mixing. Heat with mixing to 70°C and add individually the remaining ingredients of Part B. Combine the ingredients of Part A with mixing and heat to 70°C. Add Part A to Part B with mixing and cool to 40°C. Add Part C with mixing and cool to desired fill temperature.
pH 7.0+ .5

#29
(Face, Body)
(Mild Cationic, Low Solids)

Part A

INCROQUAT BEHENYL TMS	1.17
POLAWAX	1.00
CRODACOL S-95	.33
CRODAMOL PMP	1.00
CRODAMOL PTC	.67
Carnation Mineral Oil	1.00
Snow White Petrolatum	2.00
Dimethicone 350cs (200fl)	.50

Part B

Water, deionized	82.33
Glycerin	8.00

Part C

GERMABEN II	1.00
HYDROTRITICUM 2000	1.00

Combine ingredients of Part A with mixing and heat to 75°C. Combine ingredients of Part B with mixing and heat to 75°C. Add Part B to Part A with good mixing. Continue mixing and cool to 45°C. Add Part C with mixing and cool to desired fill temperature.

#30
(Behenyl Hand)

Part A	
INCROMINE BB	3.0
CRODACID B	2.5
CRODAMOL PMP	20.0
DOW SF-200 - 200cps	3.0
Part B	
Deionized Water	68.5
Part C	
GERMABEN II	1.0
Part D	
Fragrance	2.0

Combine ingredients of Part A with mixing and heat to 85-90°C. Heat Part B to 85-90°C. Add Part B to Part A with good mixing and cool to 45°C. Add Part C with mixing and cool to 40°C. Add Part D with mixing and cool to desired fill temperature.

#31
(Hand, Light Conditioning)

Water Phase:	
GLUCQUAT 100	1.0
Deionized water	84.0
Oil Phase:	
GLUCATE SS	0.8
GLUCAMATE SSE-20	1.2
ACETULAN	2.0
PROMULGEN D	3.0
Glyceryl Monostearate (neutral)	0.5

Mineral oil, 70 vis.	7.5
Perfume and preservative	q.s.

Dissolve GLUCQUAT 100 in deionized water, and heat to 70°C. Combine oil phase ingredients, and heat to 70°C with propeller agitation. Slowly add water phase to oil phase, and mix until uniform. Cool to room temperature with mixing.

#32

(Catonic Hand)

Oil Phase:	
AMERCHOL L-101®	5.0
SOLULAN® 98	2.0
CETAL	1.0
Glyceryl Stearate (and) PEG-100 Stearate	4.0
Water Phase:	
Part A	
QUATRISOFT ™ POLYMER LM-200	0.5
Water	19.5
Part B	
Steapyrium Chloride	0.1
Glycerin	2.0
Water	65.9
Preservative and Perfume	q.s.

Add QUATRISOFT ™ POLYMER LM-200 to the water (water phase, part A). Mix until thoroughly dispersed, then heat to 45°-50°C. Mix until clear and uniform. Add water phase, part A to water phase, part B with mixing while heating to 70°C. Heat oil phase to 70°C. Add water phase at 70°C to oil phase at 70°C while mixing. Cool to 35°C.

#33

(Enriched Hand)

Water Phase:	
UCARE Polymer JR-125	0.25
Propylene glycol	4.80
Triethanolamine (99%)	0.95
Deionized water	84.00

Oil Phase:

AMERCHOL C	0.50
CETAL	0.40
PROMYR	2.40
Stearic Acid, xxx	2.90
Mineral Oil, 70 vis.	2.40
Glyceryl Stearate	1.00
Myristyl Myristate	0.40
Perfume and preservative	q.s.

Heat oil phase to 70°C. Separately, add the UCARE Polymer JR-125 to the water. When hydrated, add the remaining water soluble ingredients and heat to 70°C. Add the water phase to the oil phase with vigorous stirring. Continue to mix to 35°C and pour.

#34

(Hand, Heavy Viscosity)

Oil Phase:

AMERLATE® P	2.0
Stearyl alcohol	2.0
Mineral oil, 70 vis.	4.0
Propylene glycol monostearate	1.5
Polyethylene glycol 1500 monostearate	1.0

Water Phase:

CARBOPOL 941	0.2
Triethanolamine, 10% in water	2.0
Sorbitol	3.5
Water	83.8
Perfume and Preservative	q.s.

Disperse Carbopol thoroughly in water at 85°C. Add remaining ingredients of water phase. Add water to oil phase at 85°C with good stirring. Cool while stirring to 45°C. Add perfume, continue stirring to 30°C.

To reduce viscosity, replace part of stearyl alcohol with cetyl alcohol. To reduce tack, replace sorbitol with GLUCAM E-20.

#35
(Hand, Emollient)

Oil Phase:	
AMERCHOL ® 400	1.0
SOLULAN® 5	1.0
Stearic acid, xxx	3.0
Glyceryl monostearate, neut.	2.0
Mineral oil, 70 vis.	9.0
Water Phase:	
Water	78.0
Propylene glycol	5.0
Triethanolamine	1.0
Perfume and Preservative	q.s.

Add the water phase at 85°C to the oil phase at 85°C while mixing. Stir and cool to 45°C. Add perfume, stir to 30°C.

To improve lubricity, replace part of mineral oil with AMERLATE P. To reduce oiliness, replace part of mineral oil with ACETULAN and isopropyl myristate.

#36
(Hand, Medium Viscosity)

Oil Phase:	
SOLULAN® 98	2.0
SOLULAN® 5	1.0
ARLACEL 165	4.0
Cetyl alcohol	1.0
Mineral oil, 70 vis.	4.0
Water Phase:	
EMCOL E 607S	0.1
Glycerine	2.0
Water	85.9
Perfume and Preservative	q.s.

Add the water phase at 75°C to the oil phase at 75°C while stirring. Stir and cool to 45°C. Add perfume, stir to 30°C.

To increase substantivity, increase Emcol 607S. To reduce tack, replace glycerine with GLUCAM E-20. To reduce viscosity, replace part of cetyl alcohol with myristyl alcohol. To increase viscosity, replace part of cetyl alcohol with stearyl alcohol.

#37
(Hand, Medium Viscosity)

Oil Phase:	
MODULAN®	2.0
Cetyl alcohol	2.0
Mineral oil, 70 vis.	10.0
BRIJ 76	2.0
Water Phase:	
Water	76.8
CARBOPOL 941	0.2
GLUCAM® E-20	5.0
Triethanolamine, 10% in water	2.0
Perfume and Preservative	q.s.

Disperse Carbopol in water at 85°C with high speed mixing. Add triethanolamine solution and GLUCAM E-20. Add water to oil phase at 85°C with good mixing. Cool with mixing to 45°C, add perfume oil, cool while mixing to 30°C.

To increase viscosity, replace part of cetyl alcohol with stearyl alcohol. To decrease viscosity, replace part of cetyl alcohol with myristyl alcohol. To improve lubricity, replace part of mineral oil with AMERLATE P. To add body replace part of mineral oil with PPG-36 oleate.

#38
(Hand, Medium Viscosity)

Oil Phase:	
SOLULAN® 5	0.5
Mineral oil, 70 vis.	2.0
Stearic acid, xxx	5.0
Cetyl alcohol	1.0
Glyceryl monostearate, self-emulsifying	1.5

Water Phase:

Triethanolamine	1.0
Propylene glycol	3.5
Water	85.5
Perfume and Preservative	q.s.

Heat both phases to 85°C. Add water to oil with good stirring. Cool while stirring to 45°C. Add perfume, continue stirring to 30°C.

To increase gloss, replace part of stearic acid with AMERLATE LFA. To decrease viscosity, replace part of cetyl alcohol with myristyl alcohol. To increase viscosity, replace part of cetyl alcohol with stearyl alcohol. To reduce tack of residual feel, replace propylene glycol with GLUCAM E-20 and part of mineral oil with AMERLATE P.

#39

(Hand, Low Viscosity)

Oil Phase:

AMEROXOL® OE-10	0.3
AMERCHOL® L-500	1.0
Beeswax	2.0
Spermwax	2.0
Mineral oil, 70 vis.	16.0
Sorbitan monostearate	2.4

Water Phase:

CARBOPOL 941	0.2
Triethanolamine, 10% in water	2.0
Polysorbate 60	3.6
COSMERLAC	0.5
Water	70.0
Perfume and Preservative	q.s.

Disperse Carbopol in water at 85°C with high speed mixing. Add triethanolamine solution, Polysorbate 60 and Cosmerlac with good dispersion. Add water to oil phase at 85°C with good mixing, cool while stirring to 45°C, add perfume, stir to 30°C.

To improve slip, replace beeswax with cetyl alcohol. GLUCATE SS and GLUCAMATE SSE-20 can function as alternates to the sorbitan monostearate/polysorbate 60 emulsifiers, but will require rebalancing.

#40

(Hand, Moderately, Heavy)

Oil Phase:	%
GLUCATE® SS	1.0
ACETULAN®	2.0
Cetyl alcohol	2.0
Glyceryl monostearate, neut.	0.5
Sesame oil	10.0
Water Phase:	
GLUCAMATE® SSE-20	3.0
GLUCAM® E-20	5.0
Water	76.5
Perfume and Preservative	q.s.

Add the water phase at 80°C to the oil phase at 80°C while mixing. Stir and cool to 45°C. Add perfume, stir to 35°C.

To reduce viscosity, replace part of cetyl alcohol with myristyl alcohol. Other natural oils such as peanut, avocado, corn, etc. can replace sesame oil in whole or in part, but may require emulsifier rebalancing.

#41

(Hand, Pearlescent)

Oil Phase:	
AMERCHOL® L-99	4.0
Polysorbate 80	1.0
Stearic acid, xxx	4.0
Paraffin	1.3
Glyceryl monostearate, neut.	2.0
SOLULAN® 25	2.0

Water Phase:

Propylene glycol	5.0
Albagel	0.5
Water	80.2
Perfume and Preservative	q.s.

Disperse Albagel in water at 85°C with high speed mixing. Add water phase to oil phase at 85°C with good mixing. Stir while cooling to 45°C. Add perfume, continue stirring to 30°C.

To increase body and reduce tack, replace propylene glycol with GLUCAM E-20. To improve slip, replace paraffin with mixture of AMERLATE P and cetyl alcohol. To impart satiny feel, replace part of stearic acid with PPG-36 oleate.

#42

(Hand, Protein)

Part A

Stearic Acid (Triple Pressed)	3.0
Mineral Oil, Light	5.0
MACKESTER TD-88	2.0

Part B

MACKPRO NLP	2.0
TEA	0.3
Propylene Glycol	6.0
MACKSTAT DM	q.s.
Water, Dye, Fragrance qs to	100.0

Heat parts A and B separately to 70 degrees C. Add part A to part B. Cool and fill at 30 degrees C.

#43

(Hand, Banana)

Water	568
Carbomer 934	2
GMS-SE	4
LIPOVOL A	16
ROSSWAX 573	4

COCONUT OIL #76	16
ROSS JOJOBA OIL	4
TEA	4
GERMABEN II	6
Fragrance® GK-17	q.s.

Heat the water to 60 C under agitation and slowly add the Carbomer 934. When the water is fully mixed add the 573, GMS, LIPOVOL A, Coconut Oil and Jojoba Oil that have been heated to 65 C in separate kettle. As soon as the Oil Phase has been mixed well, add the Germaben II and then the TEA under high agitation, then the fragrance. Cool to 55 C for filling.

#44
(Hand, Apricot)

Water	568
Carbomer 934	2
GMS-SE	4
LIPOVOL P	16
ROSSWAX 573	4
COCONUT OIL #76	16
ROSS JOJOBA OIL	4
TEA	4
GERMABEN II	6
Fragrance	q.s.

Heat the water to 60 C under agitation and slowly add the Carbomer 934. When the water is fully mixed, add the 573, GMS, Apricot Oil, Coconut Oil and Jojoba Oil that have been heated to 65 C in a separate kettle. As soon as the Oil Phase has been mixed well, add to the Water Phase with agitation. When fully mixed, add the Germaben II and then the TEA under high agitation, then fragrance. Cool to 55 C for filling.

#45
(Hand, Strawberry)

Water	568
Carbomer 934	2
GMS-SE	4
LIPOVOL P	16

ROSSWAX 573	4
COCONUT OIL #76	16
ROSS JOJOBA OIL	4
TEA	4
GERMABEN II	6
Fragrance	q.s.

Heat the water to 60 C under agitation and slowly add the Carbomer 934. When the water is fully mixed, add the 573, GMS, Apricot Oil, Coconut Oil and Jojoba Oil that have been heated to 65 C in a separate kettle. As soon as the oil phase has been mixed well, add the Germaben II, the fragrance, and then the TEA under high agitation. Cool to 55 C for filling.

#46

(Hand, Peach)

Water	568.0
Carbomer 934	2.0
ROSSWAX 573	4.0
GMS-SE	4.0
LIPOVOL ALM	16.0
COCONUT OIL #76	16.0
ROSS JOJOBA OIL	4.0
TEA	4.0
GERMABEN II	6.0
Fragrance	q.s.

Heat the water to 60 C under agitation and slowly add the Carbomer 934. When the water is fully mixed add the 573, GMS, Almond Oil, Coconut Oil, and Jojoba Oil that have been heated to 65 C in a separate kettle. As soon as the Oil Phase has been mixed well, add the Germaben II, the Fragrance, and then the TEA under high agitation. Cool to 55 C for filling.

#47

(Hand and Body)

A	VEEGUM	1.00
	CMC 7MF	0.15
	Water	80.75
	DOW CORNING ANTIFOAM FG-10 EMULSION	0.10

B	MARCOL 130	5.00
	AMERCHOL L-101	4.00
	Stearic acid xxx	3.00
	ARLACEL 165	4.00
	LANTROL	2.00
	Preservative	q.s.

Blend VEEGUM and CMC. Slowly add to the water, while agitating at maximum available shear. Continue mixing until smooth. Add antifoam at a slow mixing speed. Heat A to 70°C and B to 75°C. Add B to A and mix until cool. Pour off at 40°C.

Consistency: Medium viscosity lotion.
Suggested Packaging: Squeeze or pump bottle.

#48
(Hand and Body)

A	VEEGUM	1.5
	CMC 7MF	0.5
	Water	67.9
	Glycerin	6.0
	Allantoin	0.1
B	CARNATION WHITE MINERAL OIL	5.0
	Petrolatum	4.0
	ACETULAN	6.0
	AMERCHOL L-101	4.0
	ARLACEL 165	5.0
	Preservative	q.s.

Blend VEEGUM and CMC. Slowly add to the water, while agitating at maximum available shear. Continue mixing until smooth. Add the glycerin and allantoin and heat A to 70-75°C. Heat B to 70-75°C. Add B to A and mix to room temperature.

Consistency: Medium viscosity lotion.
Suggested Packaging: Squeeze or pump bottle.

#49

(Hand & Body, High Oil)

Part A	
INCROQUAT BEHENYL TMS	1.50
CRODAMOL PMP	10.00
CRILL 6	0.75
FLUILAN	0.50
Part B	
Water, deionized	84.45
INCROMECTANT LAMEA	1.00
CARBOPOL 941	0.40
TEA 99%	0.40
Part C	
GERMABEN II	1.00

Dust in the Carbopol 941 of Part B into the water with good mixing and allow to hydrate. Add other ingredients of Part B, except for the TEA with mixing and heat to 75-80°C. At 75-80°C, add the TEA. Heat to 80°C. Combine ingredients of Part A with mixing and heat to 80°C. Add Part A to Part B with good mixing. Continue mixing and cool to 45°C. Add Part C with mixing and cool to desired fill temperature. Adjust pH with a 10% TEA solution to 5.9.

#50

(Hand and Body, Lotion Medium Viscosity)

Oil Phase:	
AMERCHIOL L-101®	6.0
MODULAN®	2.0
Stearic acid, xxx	2.0
Glyceryl monostearate, acid stable	2.0
Water Phase:	
Propylene glycol	5.0
Sodium Lauryl sulfate	1.0
VEEGUM	0.5
Water	81.5
Perfume and Preservative	q.s.

Disperse Veegum in water and hold at 90°C while stirring for one hour. Add remaining water phase ingredients and add the water phase at 85°C to the oil phase at 85°C while mixing. Mix while cooling to 45°C. Add the perfume. Continue mixing and cool to 30°C.

To improve body, replace propylene glycol with GLUCAM P-10. To increase lubricity, replace stearic acid with mixture of AMERLATE P and AMERLATE LFA.

#51

(Hand and Body)

A	VEEGUM® PRO	2.00
	Water	70.75
	Glycerin	6.00
B	MARCOL 130	10.00
	Petrolatum	4.00
	ARLACEL 165	5.00
	SYNCHROWAX AW1-C	1.25
C	Allantoin	1.00
	Preservative	q.s.

Heat the water to 70 to 75°C, then slowly add the VEEGUM PRO while agitating at maximum available shear. Mix until smooth. Add glycerine and mix until uniform. Heat B to 75 to 80°C. Add B to A and mix until cool. Add C and mix until uniform.

Consistency: Medium viscosity lotion.
Suggested Packaging: Squeeze or pump bottle.

#52

(Hand and Body)

Part 1

Water	78.6
Carbomer 934	.2

Part 2

MODULAN	1.6
IPP	3.8
AMERCHOL L-101	.8
GMS SE	2.1
ROSSWAX 63-0412	4.0
IPM	4.0
Jojoba Oil	1.6

Part 3

GERMABEN IIE	1.0

Part 4

Fragrance	q.s.

Part 5

Triethanolamine	2.3

Part A

Disperse the carbomer 934 in the water phase in a stainless steel kettle.

Part B

In a separate heated kettle, heat the oil phase until all ingredients are melted. When everything is melted add the oil phase to the water phase. When everything is blended add the preservative, the fragrance and the Triethanolamine with increased agitation. Cool to room temperature and package.

#53

(Hand and Body, Non-greasy)

Part A

PHOSPHOLIPID EFA	4.00
Water	83.00

Part B

Steareth-2	2.00
Light Mineral Oil	4.00
Cetearyl Alcohol	3.00
Octydodecyl Myristate	2.50
Dimethicone (100cS)	1.50

Combine ingredients in both phases separately and heat to 65°C. Homogenize (B) into (A) with continued heating until sufficiently mixed. Stir-cool to 40°C. Add fragrance, color, and preservative as needed and fill.

#54
(Hand, Body, Low Viscosity)

Oil Phase:	
GLUCATE® SS	1.0
GLUCAMATE® SSE-20	1.5
MODULAN®	2.0
Stearic acid, xxx	2.0
Mineral Oil, 70 vis.	6.0
Water Phase:	
GLUCAM® E-20	5.0
Water	82.5
Perfume and Preservative	q.s.

Add the water phase at 85°C to the oil phase at 85°C while mixing. Stir and cool to 45°C. Add perfume, stir to 30°C.

Formula is well balanced and modifications of oil phase will require adjustment of the emulsifier ratio and concentrations. For example- replacement of mineral oil with vegetable oils.

#55
(Hand & Body, High Viscosity)

Oil Phase:	
GLUCATE® SS	1.5
GLUCAMATE® SSE-20	1.5
MODULAN®	1.0
Mineral oil, 70 vis.	4.0
Glyceryl monostearate, neut.	2.0
Water Phase:	
EMCOL E-607S	1.0
Glycerine	5.0
METHOCEL 65HG	0.2

Water	83.8
Perfume and Preservative	q.s.

Disperse the Methocel in water using high speed mixing. When even with no lumps, add remaining ingredients of the water phase. Add the water phase at 80°C to the oil phase at 80°C while mixing. Stir and cool to 45°C. Add perfume, stir to 30°C.

To reduce viscosity, replace mineral oil with a mixture of AMERLATE P and isopropyl myristate. Replace glycerine with GLUCAM E-10.

#56

(Moisturizing)

Oil Phase:

AMERLATE P	0.5
Stearic Acid	3.0
Glyceryl Stearate	2.0

Water Phase:

GLUCAM E-20	5.0
Triethanolamine	1.0
Water	83.7
BIOCARE POLYMER HA-24	3.8
GERMABEN IIE	1.0

Add BioCare Polymer HA-24 to water at 25°C. Mix until thoroughly dispersed. Heat to 45-50°C if necessary. When dispersed, add the GLUCAM E-20 and triethanolamine and heat to 85°C. Add the water phase at 85°C to the oil phase at 85°C with good stirring. Add the preservative Germaben IEE at 75°C. Continue to mix to room temperature with thorough agitation.

#57

(Moisturizing)

Water Phase:

KYTAMER ™ PC	1.0
GLUCAMATE® SSE-20	1.5
Deionized Water	82.0

Oil Phase:

GLUCATE® SS	1.5
PROMULGEN® G	4.0
Mineral Oil	10.0
Perfume and Preservative	q.s.

Disperse KYTAMER ™ PC in water at room temperature with high speed agitation. When completely dispersed heat to 75°C with continuous mixing until clear and uniform. Maintain temperature at 75°C and add GLUCAMATE® SSE-20. Heat oil phase to 75°C. Add the water phase at 75°C to oil phase at 75°C with good agitation. Continue mixing while slowly cooling to room temperature. Add perfume below 50°C.

#58

(Moisturizing)

Oil Phase:

PROMULGEN® D	5.0
Mineral oil	4.0
CETAL	2.0
AMEROXOL® OE-2	1.0
GLUCAMATE® SSE-20	2.0
Dimethicone	1.0
GLUCAM® E-20 DISTEARATE	1.0

Water Phase:

GLUCATE® SS	2.0
Deionized water	81.0
BIOCARE® SA	1.0
Perfume and preservative	q.s.

Heat the oil phase to 80°C, heat water phase minus the BioCare® SA to 80°C. Add water to oil at 80°C, add perfume and BioCare® SA below 35°C. Continue mixing with moderate agitation while cooling to room temperature.

#59

(Pourable Moisturizing)

Part I	
Deionized Water	84.3
MONAQUAT P-TS	2.0
Glycerin (99%)	3.0
PEG 12	2.0
Part II	
Light Mineral Oil	3.0
Isopropyl Isostearate	2.0
Cetyl Alcohol (95%)	2.0
Dimethicone (100 C.S.)	0.2
Propylene Glycol Monostearate (Pure)	1.5

Heat Part I to 65°C, with mixing, until clear. Heat Part II to 65°C, with mixing. Slowly add Part II to Part I with efficient mixing. Remove heat after 5 minutes.Cool slowly. When the temperature drops to the 45° -40°C range the product will thicken somewhat and the propeller rotational speed will slow down. Increase the speed to ensure thorough mixing. Add fragrance, coloring or preservative as required. Cool to 27°C or below and fill.

#60

(W/O Moisturizing)

A	VEEGUM	1.3
	Water	55.7
	Magnesium sulphate	0.5
B	Mineral oil, light	9.0
	POLYSYNLANE	10.0
	NIMLESTEROL D	7.5
	AMERCHOL L-101	9.0
	Sorbitol, 70% soln.	5.0
	WITCAMIDE 511	2.0
	Preservative	q.s.

Add the VEEGUM to the water slowly, agitating with maximum available shear until smooth. Add the magnesium sulphate and mix until smooth. Blend B well and add A to B; mix until smooth and uniform.

Consistency/Suggested Packaging: medium viscosity lotion/bottle.

#61

(Intensive Moisturizing)

Part A	
CRODACOL C-70	1.0
CRODALAN LA	1.0
Glyceryl Monostearate	1.0
CARNATION MINERAL OIL	5.0
Stearic Acid XXX	2.0
SILICONE FLUID SP96-50	1.0
Part B	
Water, deionized	73.4
VEEGUM HV	.5
GERMABEN II	1.0
Glycerin	10.0
HAMPENE Na2	.1
TEA 99%	1.0
D&C Yellow #10	q.s.
Part C	
CARBOPOL 934 (2.5% aqueous slurry)	3.0

Combine the water and Veegum of Part B while mixing and heat to 75°C. Add the remaining ingredients of Part B individually with mixing. Combine ingredients of Part A with mixing and heat to 75°C. Add Part B to Part A with good mixing and cool to 60°C. Add Part C with mixing and cool to desired fill temperature.

#62

(O/W Ultra Moisturizing)

This creamy oil-in-water emulsion is thickened and stabilized with a combination of VEEGUM *Ultra* and Carbomer.The well known humectant glycerin provides the moisturizing function. VEEGUM *Ultra* also enhances the whiteness and brightness of the emulsion and helps adjust the pH to approximate that of the skin. The lotion spreads easily and is rapidly absorbed leaving the skin moist and supple.

A	VEEGUM® *Ultra*	0.15
	Carbomer 980	0.15
	Deionized Water	73.70
B	Glycerin	5.00
C	Mineral Oil (and) Lanolin Alcohol	4.00
	Cetyl alcohol	2.00
	Isopropyl Palmitate	2.00
	Hydrogenated Polyisobutene	5.00
	Isopropyl Myristate	3.00
	Sorbitan Palmitate	1.20
	Polysorbate 40	3.80
D	Preservative, Fragrance	q.s.
	Triethanolamine to pH 6.0	q.s.

Dry blend VEEGUM *Ultra* and Carbomer and add them slowly to the water while stirring with a propeller mixer at 700 rpm. Increase the mixer speed to 1500-1700 rpm and continue mixing for 30 minutes. Add B and mix 5 minutes. Mix C ingredients and heat to 50°C. Heat A and B mixture to 50°C. Add C to A and B and mix at 50°C and 1500-1700 rpm for 10 minutes.Slow the mixer to 1000 rpm while cooling to 30°C. Add D and mix until uniform.

Properties:
Viscosity - 2200-2800 cps
pH - 6.0 ± 0.2
Color - White, Bright

#63
(Super Moisturizing)

A	VEEGUM	1.0
	RHODIGEL	0.5
	Deionized Water	74.5
B	Sodium PCA	3.0
	Glycerine	5.0

C	Hydrogenated Polyisobutene	4.0
	Mineral Oil (and) Lanolin Alcohol	3.0
	Cetyl Alcohol	2.0
	Isopropyl Myristate	2.0
	Sorbitan Palmitate	1.2
	Polysorbate 40	3.8
D	Citric Acid to pH 5.5	q.s.
	Preservative, Dye, Fragrance	q.s.

Dry blend VEEGUM and RHODIGEL and add to the water, mixing with maximum available shear until smooth and uniform. Add B ingredients and mix until dissolved. Mix C ingredients and heat to 50°C until a uniform clear mixture is obtained. Add C to (A + B) with high speed mixing. Avoid incorporating air. Cool with continuous stirring to 30°C and add D.
CONSISTENCY: Medium Viscosity Lotion (Viscosity - 1900-2400 cps; Brookfield Model LVT, spindle 4 at 60 rpm, measured at RT after 30 days aging.)
SUGGESTED PACKAGING: Plastic squeeze bottle or pump.

#64

(Depilatory)

A	VEEGUM HS	1
	Water	74
B	Propylene glycol	5
C	AMERCHOL L-101	5
	SOLULAN 98	2
	ARLACEL 165	2
D	Calcium thioglycolate	5
	Calcium hydroxide	6
	Preservative	q.s.

Slowly add VEEGUM HS to the water, while agitating maximum available shear. Continue mixing until smooth. Add B to A and heat to 75°C. Heat C to 70°C. Add C to A/B with stirring. Cool to 45°C. Add calcium thioglycolate and stir. Add the calcium hydroxide and stir until cool and uniform.

Consistency: Viscous lotion.
Suggested Packaging: Squeeze bottle or tube.

Overnight Moisturizer

Part A	
PHOSPHOLIPID EFA	4.00
PEG-32	2.00
Glycerin	2.00
Water	73.00
Part B	
Steareth-2	2.50
Cetearyl Alcohol	4.00
Cetyl Palmitate	4.00
Myristyl Myristate	4.00
Isopropyl Palmitate	3.00
Dimethicone (100cS)	1.50

Blend and heat both phases separately to 70°c. Homogenize (B) into (A) with continued heat for an appropriate time while avoiding aeration. Stir-cool to 45°C, then add fragrance, coloring, or preservative as required and fill.

Essential skin Moisturizer

(Gel)

Deionized water	94.5
CELLOSIZE® POLYMER PCG-10	0.5
GLUCAM® E-10	2.0
Glycerin	2.0
BIOCARE® SA	1.0
Preservative and perfume	q.s.

Disperse CELLOSIZE® POLYMER PCG-10 in water; facilitate mixing with gentle heating. When solution is clear, add GLUCAM® E-10 and glycerin and cool to room temperature. Add BioCare® SA and perfume below 35°C.

Multi-Protective Skin Moisturizer

(Cationic)

Part A	
Cetyl Alcohol	2.00
DRAKEOL 7	3.00
Petrolatum	1.00
Tridecyl Neopentanoate	2.50
ABIL B8852	1.00
CERASYNT 945	1.00
DOW CORNING 200 FLUID	0.20
Tocopheryl Acetate (Vitamin E Acetate)	0.20
BRIJ 721	1.00
Phase B	
Water	70.90
MONOQUAT P-TS	2.00
Allantoin	0.50
Aloe Vera Gel 1:1	5.00
CELQUAT SC-240	0.50
Propylene Glycol	4.00
DRY FLO-C	4.00
Phase C	
GERMABEN II-E	1.00
Phase D	
Fragrance	0.20

Heat water, Monoquat and Allantoin to 50°C. Add Celquat SC-240, disperse thoroughly and heat to 80°C. Prepare propylene glycol and Dry Flo-C slurry and add to water phase. Mix Phase B and heat to 80°C. Add Phase B to Phase A at 80°C and mix for 15 minutes. Cool to 35°C and add Phase C and Phase D to it. Cool to room temperature and homogenize.

Skin Conditioning Mousse Concentrate

(Aerosol)

Phase A	
SOLULAN® 16	1.5
GLUCAM® P-10	1.5
SOLULAN® 98	2.0

Phase B	
Deionized Water	78.5
QUATRISOFT ™ POLYMER LM-200	0.5
Preservatives	1.0
Phase C	
SD Alcohol 40	15.0

Concentrate: Add QUATRISOFT ™ POLYMER LM-200 to agitating water at 25°C. Heat to 70°C and mix until dissolved. Add preservatives to complete phase B. In a separate container add phase A ingredients and heat to 70°C with agitation. Add phase B to A and mix until uniform. Cool to 40°C and add phase C. Cool to 25°C when uniform.

Aerosol Fill: Fill aluminum mousse can and charge with A-46 Propellant using 90% product and 10% propellant.

Liquid Cold Cream

A	VEEGUM	1.0
	Water	69.0
B	WAXENOL 821 S.B.	1.5
	CRODAMOL SS	1.5
	MARCOL 130	20.0
	ARLACEL 40	3.5
	TWEEN 60	3.5
	Preservative	q.s.

Slowly add VEEGUM to the water, while agitating at maximum available shear. Continue mixing until smooth. Heat A to 75°C. Heat B to 80°C. Add B to A and mix until cool.
Consistency: Pourable lotion.
Suggested Packaging: Squeeze or pump container.

Airy Skin Conditioning Mousse

(Concentrate)

QUATRISOFT ™ POLYMER LM-200	1.0
Propylene Glycol	2.0
Ethanol SD-40	15.0

Deionized Water	82.0
Preservative and Perfume	q.s.

Mix ethanol with water at room temperature. Add QUATRISOFT ™ POLYMER LM-200 and other ingredients with water/ethanol mixture using rapid stirring at room temperature until polymer is completely dissolved.

Aerosol: Fill Aluminum mousse can and charge with A-46 Propellant using a weight ratio of 100 parts of product to 20 parts of propellant.

Clear Collagen Facial Conditioner

(Liquid)

Water, deionized	89.00
CLEARCOL	5.00
RETICUSOL	1.00
CROTEIN CAA SF	1.00
INCROMECTANT AQ	1.50
PVP K-90	1.00
CMC 7MF	.50
GERMABEN II	1.00
Triethanolamine (99%)	q.s.

First dissolve the CLEARCOL in water. Heat gently to not more than 30°C (Warning: Soluble Collagen denatures above 35°C) and add PVP K-90 and CMC 7MF. Add the remaining ingredients, then adjust pH to 6.5 with 10% solution of Triethanolamine (99%) to form a clear, colorless solution.

Skin Guardian

Phase A	
Water	77.500
CARBOPOL 941	0.300
HAMPENE Na3T	0.300
Triethanolamine	0.500
Phase B	
CARBOWAX 335	2.000
LIPONIC EG-1	1.500
VOLPO 20	3.500

CROVOL A-70	0.500
CRODESTA F-160	1.300
Allantoin	0.500
GERMABEN II	1.000
Phase C	
DOW CORNING 190	2.000
Butylene glycol	2.000
Panthenol (Dexpanthenol)	0.100
Retinyl Palmitate (Vitamin A Palmitate)	0.100
Squalane	0.200
BHT	0.200
VOLPO 10	2.000
Octyl Methoxycinnamate	0.100
Glycoceramides (and) Phospholipids (and) Cholesterol (Glycosomes)	0.100
Phase D	
CROMOIST HY	1.000
CROTEIN SPA	3.000
Phase E	
Triethanolamine, 99%	0.250
Phase F	
FD&C Red #4, 1% Solution	0.025
FD&C Yellow #5, 1% Solution	0.025

Dust Carbopol 941 into cold water under moderate agitation. Let mix until completely hydrated (30 minutes). Add Hampene Na3T. Mix until clear. Neutralize Carbopol with triethanolamine. Add the ingredients fro Phase B to Phase A in the order listed, mixing after each addition until the batch is uniform. Warm batch to 60°C to mix in Crodesta F-160, Allantoin, and Germaben II. Maintain 60°C for addition of Phase C. While warming Phase B, prepare Phase C in a separate vessel. Add ingredients sequentially, mixing after each addition and warm mixture to 63°C. When clear and at 63°C, add Phase C to batch slowly with mixing. Mix until uniform. Let cool with mixing to 40°C. Add Phase D ingredients sequentially. Add Phase E and Phase F at room temperature. Adjust pH to 7.2.

Chapter VII

MOUTH PREPARATIONS

Toothpaste

#1

A	VEEGUM	1.0
	Water	18.5
B	CMC 7HF	0.5
	Glycerin	30.0
C	Dicalcium phosphate	47.0
D	Flavor	1.0
E	Sodium lauryl sulfate	2.0
	Preservative	q.s.

Slowly add VEEGUM to the water, while agitating at maximum available shear. Continue mixing until smooth. Wet the CMC with glycerin. Slowly add to A with agitation. Slowly add C with agitation. Add D and mix. Slowly add E with just enough mixing to get a smooth batch.

Consistency: Thick paste.
Suggested Packaging: Tube.

#2
(Fluoride)

A	VEEGUM	1.00
	CMC 7MF	0.70
	Water	20.25
B	Glycerin	12.50
	Sorbitol 70%	12.50
C	Stannous fluoride	0.40
	Saccharin	0.15
	Calcium pyrophosphate	45.00
D	Flavor	1.00
E	HAMPOSYL L-30	6.50
	Preservative	q.s.

Blend VEEGUM and CMC. Slowly add to the water, while agitating at maximum available shear. Continue mixing until smooth. Add B slowly and mix until smooth. Add C ingredients in order, mixing after each addition until smooth and uniform. Add D and E and mix until smooth. Avoid incorporation of air.

Consistency: thick paste.
Suggested Packaging: Tube.

#3
(Fluoride)

		Gel	Gel Pump
A	VEEGUM	1.50	0.75
	Water	24.50	19.10
B	Sorbitol 70%	36.50	50.00
C	Glycerin	10.00	10.00
	CMC 7MF	-	1.00

D	SYLOID 74	24.00	13.00
	SYLOID 63	-	3.00
E	Flavor	1.20	1.00
F	Sodium fluoride	0.25	0.25
	Saccharin	0.20	0.20
	Sodium Benzoate	0.20	0.20
	MAPROFIX	1.50	1.50
	Citric Acid	0.15	-
	Color	q.s.	q.s.

Slowly add VEEGUM to the water, while agitating at maximum available shear. Continue mixing until smooth. Mix in B, followed by C (Preblend CMC into glycerin for pump). Mix until smooth. Add D, E, and F in order, mixing after each addition until smooth and uniform.

Consistency: Thick gel; Soft gel.
Suggested Packaging: Tube; Pump bottle.

#4
(Gel)

A	VEEGUM	1.00
	CMC 7MF	0.25
	Water	21.25
B	Sorbitol 70%	12.50
	Glycerin	12.50
C	Dicalcium phosphate dihydrate	50.00
D	Flavor	1.00
E	MAPROFIX 563	1.50
	Preservative	q.s.

Blend VEEGUM and CMC. slowly add to the water, while agitating at maximum available shear. Continue mixing until smooth. Add B to A while mixing. Add C and D while mixing until smooth. Add E with slow mixing. Avoid incorporation of air.

Consistency: Flowable gel.
Suggested Packaging: Plastic squeeze bottle.

Tooth Powder

#1

Precipitated Chalk (Calcium Carbonate)	1 3/4 cup
Magnesium Carbonate	1 cup
Powdered Sugar	3/4 cup
Sodium Perborate	1/2 cup
Powdered Neutral White Soap	1/4 cup
Flavor, as desired	

Put all ingredients except flavoring into mortar and rub down well. Add Flavor slowly and continue to rub well until evenly mixed.

#2

(Ammoniated)

LATHANOL LAL	3.0
Tricalcium Phosphate	87.8
Urea	3.0
Dibasic Ammonium Phosphate	5.0
Saccharin	0.2
Flavor	1

Mix dry ingredients thoroughly. Add Flavor and mix until homogenous.

Denture Cleaner

#1

A	VEEGUM	1.0
	Sodium Carboxymethylcellulose (med. visc.)	0.5
	Water	28.9
B	Saccharin	0.1
	Sodium Benzoate	1.0
C	Sorbitol (70% sol'n.)	9.0
	Glycerin	9.0

D	Dicalcium Phosphate Dihydrate	36.0
	Dicalcium Phosphate Anhydrous	12.0
E	Flavor	0.5
F	Sodium Lauryl Sulfate	2.0

Dry blend the VEEGUM and the CMC. Add to the Water slowly, agitating continually until smooth. Add (B) to (A) and mix. Blend (C) and add to (A) and (B). Blend (D) and add to the mixture. Add (E) and (F), one at a time, to other components and mix until uniform.

#2
(Tablet)

A	VEEGUM WG	5 g.
	Sodium Perborate	13 g.
	Tetrasodium Pyrophosphate Anhydrous	25 g.
	Sodium Chloride	13 g.
	Tartaric Acid	9 g.
	Sodium Phosphate Dibasic	12 g.
	Citric Acid	7 g.
	Sodium Bicarbonate	16 g.
B	Isopropyl Alcohol	25 g.
C	VEEGUM WG	2 g.

Granulate (A) with (B). Pass through a No. 10 mesh screen. Dry the granulation 1 hour @ 105°C. and pass through a No. 16 mesh screen. Dry blend with (C) and compress.

Directions for Use: Add one tablet to a glass of hot water. Soak dentures in solution one-half hour or overnight and rinse.

Mouthwash

#1
(Clear, Fluid Liquid)

PLURONIC F-108	1.000
Water	81.761
Alcohol (Ethanol 95%)	17.000

Sodium Saccharin	0.150
Spearmint Oil	0.040
Menthol	0.040
Cinnamon Oil	0.008
Dye	0.001

Weigh out Water, Alcohol and PLURONIC in suitable vessel. Mix gently until homogenous. Add Flavors, Color, and other minor ingredients and mix gently five minutes or until homogenous. Transfer to suitable containers. Amounts and ratios of flavors may be varied, depending upon consumer preference.

#2

(Zinc Chloride)

Zinc Chloride	1.00
Menthol	0.50
Oil of Cinnamon	1.30
Oil of cloves	0.50
Solution of Formaldehyde	0.50
Saccharin	0.40
Naphtol Yellow S	0.24
Alcohol	45.00
Talc	15.00
Diluted Hydrochloric Acid	1.00
Distilled Water, to make	1000.00

Dissolve the Zinc Chloride in a solution of the dilute Hydrochloric. Acid and 25 cc. of Distilled Water, and add this to 800 cc. of Distilled Water. Dissolve the Oil of Cinnamon, Oil of cloves, Menthol, Solution of Formaldehyde and Saccharin in 45 cc. of Alcohol, and mix this with 15 g. of talc. Add to this, with constant stirring, the previously prepared Zinc chloride solution, shake resulting mixture occasionally during 24 hours, and filter. Add Distilled Water to make one liter, and add a suitable color.

Mouthspray Refresher

Fungitex R	0.10
Saccharin	0.50
Peppermint Oil	0.50

Cinnamon Oil	0.25
Water	5.00
Glycerine	10.00
Alcohol #38/B	83.65

Mix all ingredients together until uniform. fill spray-type bottles with this solution.

Chapter VIII

PERFUMES AND COLOGNES

Bergamot, Essence
(Natural) No. 1

1.	Bergamot, Oil	300
2.	Limonene	300
3.	Linalool	60
4.	Linalyl Acetate	300
5.	Terpinyl Acetate	40

Bergamot, Essence
(Natural) No. 2

1.	Bergamot, Oil	430
2.	Bois de Rose, Oil	80
3.	Geranyl Acetate	30
4.	Linalyl Acetate	150
5.	Nerolin	10
6.	Petitgrain, Paraguay	20
7.	Terpineol	190
8.	Terpinyl Acetate	90

Bouquet, No. 1
(For Soap)

1.	Bergamot, Oil	325
2.	Clove, Oil	25
3.	Geranium, Oil	200

4.	Gingergrass, Oil	150
5.	Lemongrass, Oil	75
6.	Methyl Anthranilate	60
7.	Musk Xylene	40
8.	Patchouli, Oil	75
9.	Styrax	50

Bouquet, No. 2

(For Soap)

1.	Aldehyde C-10 (10% sol'n.)	25
2.	Linalool	300
3.	Linalyl Acetate	100
4.	Methyl Anthranilate	100
5.	Orange (Sweet), Oil	125
6.	Phenyl Ethyl Alcohol	350

Cananga

(For Soap)

1.	Bromostyrene	25
2.	Cedarwood, Oil	75
3.	ρ–Cresyl Methyl Ether	25
4.	Geranium Palmarosa, Oil	375
5.	Methyl anthranilate	50
6.	Musk Xylene	50
7.	Sassafras, Oil	25
8.	Terpineol	375

Lavender, Imitation

(For Soap)

1.	Benzyl Acetate	40
2.	Bergamot, Oil	125
3.	Borneol	30
4.	Coumarin	30
5.	Geranium, Oil	200
6.	Lavender, Oil	200
7.	Musk Xylene	25

8.	Patchoulii, Oil	40
9.	Rosemary, Oil	60
10.	Spike, Oil	200
11.	Thyme, Oil	50

Lavender, Sweet

1.	Bergamot, Oil	110
2.	Citral	10
3.	Coumarin	10
4.	Geranyl Acetate	20
5.	α-Ionone	20
6.	Isobornyl Acetate	50
7.	Lavender, Oil	110
8.	Linalyl Acetate	50
9.	Musk Ketone	10
10.	Pine, white Oil	10
11.	Terpinyl Acetate	10
12.	Ethyl Alcohol 95%	295
13.	Distilled Water	295

Leather

1.	Amyl Salicylate	50
2.	Balsam Peru	100
3.	Birch Tar Rectified	100
4.	Coumarin	30
5.	Methyl Salicylate	50
6.	Ethyl Alcohol 95%	335
7.	Distilled Water	335

Lilac, Imitation

#1

1.	Anisic Aldehyde	10
2.	Benzyl Acetate	30
3.	Benzyl Alcohol	40
4.	Benzyl Formate	10
5.	Benzyl Salicylate	10
6.	Cananga Oil	40

7.	Cinnamic Alcohol	100
8.	ρ-Cresyl Acetate	10
9.	Cuminic Aldehyde	10
10.	Decyl Alcohol	10
11.	Farnesol	10
12.	Heliotropin	60
13.	Hydroxycitronellal	150
14.	Isoeugenol	10
15.	Methyl Anthranilate	10
16.	Linalool	40
17.	Phenylacetaldehyde	10
18.	Phenyl Ethyl Acetate	50
19.	Phenyl Ethyl Alcohol	150
20.	Phenylpropyl Acetate	40
21.	Rose, Oil	10
22.	Terpineol	150
23.	ρ-Tolyl Aldehyde	10
24.	Tuberose, Oil	20
25.	Vanillin (10% sol'n.)	10

#2

1.	Anisic Aldehyde	140
2.	Benzyl alcohol	110
3.	Citronellol	150
4.	α-Ionone	10
5.	Musk Ketone	10
6.	Phenylacetaldehyde	10
7.	Phenyl Ethyl Alcohol (10% sol'n.)	200
8.	Terpineol	350
9.	Tuberose, Oil	10
10.	Vanillin (10% sol'n.)	10

Muguet (Lily of The Valley),

(Imitation)

#1

1.	Civet	10
2.	Jasmine, Oil	75
3.	Lime, Oil	25

4.	Linalool	150
5.	Musk Ambrette	15
6.	Rose, Oil	10
7.	Terpineol	150
8.	Ylang Ylang, Oil	25
9.	Ethyl Alcohol 95%	270
10.	Distilled Water	270

#2

1.	Aldehyde C-11 (undecylenic)	5
2.	Aldehyde C-12 (lauric)	5
3.	Aldehyde C-14 (myristic)	5
4.	Almond (Bitter), Oil (pure)	10
5.	Cassie, Oil	20
6.	Jasmine, Oil	40
7.	Orange Flowers, Oil	45
8.	Rose, Oil	10
9.	Tuberose, Oil	45
10.	Vanilla Beans, Oil	15
11.	Ethyl Alcohol 95%	400
12.	Distilled Water	400

#3

(For Soap)

1.	Benzyl Acetate	50
2.	Civet, Absolute	5
3.	Geranium Palmarosa, Oil	325
4.	Hydroxycitronellal	325
5.	Jasmine, Absolute	20
6.	Linalool	75
7.	Terpineol	75
8.	Ylang Ylang, Oil	125

Muguet (Lily of The Valley),

(Synthetic)

#1

1.	Benzyl Acetate	200
2.	Cinnamic Alcohol	200
3.	Hydroxycitronellol (10% sol'n.)	300

4.	Musk Ambrette	50
5.	Phenyl Ethyl Alcohol	100
6.	Terpineol	100
7.	Ylang Ylang, Oil	50

#2

1.	Alcohol C-9	6
2.	Alcohol C-10	1
3.	Alcohol C-11 (undecylenic)	5
4.	Aldehyde C-9	4
5.	Aldehyde C-10	3
6.	Aldehyde C-12	4
7.	Aldehyde C-16	2
8.	Cinnamyl Acetate	150
9.	Ethyl Phenyl Acetate	150
10.	Hydroxycitronellal	150
11.	Ionone	25
12.	Linalool	150
13.	Ethyl Alcohol 95%	175
14.	Distilled Water	175

Musk

1.	Ambergris	50
2.	Bergamot, Oil	250
3.	Benzyl Salicylate (10% sol'n.)	50
4.	Heliotropin	150
5.	Linalool	150
6.	Orris, Oil	50
7.	Vanillin (10% sol'n.)	150
8.	Vetiverol	150

Pomade Perfume

LANOCERIN®	10.0
GLUCATE® SS	8.0
Hydrogenated coconut oil	25.0
Petrolatum	10.0

Glyceryl monostearate pure	7.0
ACETULAN®	3.0
Microcrystalline wax	15.0
Ozokerite	5.0
CAB-O-SIL M-5	2.0
Perfume oil	15.0
Color and antioxidant	q.s.

Melt all ingredients except Cab-O-Sil M-5 and perfume oil to 80-90°C. With good stirring, add Cab-O-Sil M-5 until completely taken up. At 70-75°C, stir in perfume oil, cool to just above solidification point and pour into godets.

Perfume Stick

Coconut oil 110°	30.0
Microcrystalline wax	5.5
Ozokerite	14.0
GLUCATE® SS	7.5
Magnesium carbonate	2.0
AMERCHOL L-101®	26.0
Perfume oil	15.0
Preservative, color and antioxidant	q.s.

Heat all ingredients except perfume oil to 85-90°C. Add fragrance at 75°C. Warm slightly, mixing until uniform. Mold into sticks.

Fragrance Veil

#1

KLUCEL HF	1.0
Specially Denatured Alcohol No. 40	74.6
Natural Pearl Essence	0.1
Perfume oil	1.5
Water	18.8
GLUCAM® P-20	4.0
Color	q.s.

Sprinkle Klucel HF into alcohol with stirring until no particles remain. With stirring add natural pearl essence and remaining ingredients in order listed. Stir until homogeneous.

Mica based synthetic pearls may be substituted for the natural pearl after checking for possibility of excessive setting.

#2

Phase A:	
CARBOPOL 940, 3% aqueous dispersion	6.5
Water	51.3
ETHOMEEN C/25	0.2
Phase B:	
Perfume oil	1.5
Isostearyl alcohol	2.5
AMEROXOL® OE-10	3.0
GLUCAM® P-20	3.0
Specially Denatured Alcohol No. 40	32.0

Phase A: Add Carbopol 940 dispersion to water, then add Ethomeen C/25. Phase B: Stir all ingredients except alcohol to uniformity and then dissolve in the alcohol. Add Phase B to Phase A with moderate agitation. Stir until uniform.

Cologne

#1

Citrus or modified citrus perfume oil	5.0
GLUCAM® P-20	1.5
SOLULAN® 16	1.0
Specially Denatured Alcohol No. 40	72.5
Water	20.0
Color	q.s.

Stir all ingredients except water until homogeneous. Add water in thin stream with stirring. Age, chill and filter.

#2

1.	Beramot, Oil	200
2.	Lemon, Oil	100
3.	Musk Ambrette	1
4.	Neroli, Oil	20
5.	Orange, Oil	50
6.	Rosemary, Oil	1
7.	Ethyl Alcohol 95%	314
8.	Distilled Water	314

#3
(Stick)

LANOGENE®	3.0
AMERLATE® P	11.0
PROMYR	10.0
CETAL	15.0
AMERCHOL L-101®	10.0
MODULAN®	5.0
OHlan®	8.0
Ozokerite	18.0
Hydrogenated vegetable oil	5.0
Cocoa butter	5.0
Lanolin, anthydrous deodorized USP	5.0
Perfume oil	5.0
Color and antioxidant	q.s.

Heat all ingredients except perfume oil to 80-90°C. Add perfume oil with stirring at 70°C. Mold into sticks.

Color Base Standard

#1

1.	Distilled Water	847 ml
2.	Dyestuff	50 g
3.	Glycerin (28 Be)	100 ml
4.	Sodium Benzoate	3 g

Heat to 100 C. Dissolve well. Cool. Filter.

#2

1.	Color	10 g
2.	Ethyl Alcohol 95%	190 ml
3.	Distilled Water	800 ml

Color Mixture

		Dye	g
1.	Cherry	Blue	2.5
		Red	97.5
2.	Green	Blue	10.0
		Yellow	90.0
3.	Orange	Red	10.0
		Yellow	90.0

Cream Sachet

Phase A:	
STEARAL	5.0
ARLACEL 165	16.0
PROPAL	1.5
AMERLATE® P	2.5
GLUCATE® SS	4.0
Phase B:	
ATLAS G-2162	2.0
GLUCAM® P-20	3.0
Water	56.0
Phase C:	
Perfume oil	10.0
Perfume	q.s.

Heat Phases A&B separately to 75-80°C. Add Phase B to Phase A with stirring. cool with stirring to 60°C, add Phase C (perfume). With moderate agitation, cool to just above congealing point and fill into container.

For softer consistency, replace all or part of Stearal with Cetal. For creamier texture, replace G-2162 with Promulgen D.

Chapter IX

SHAVING PREPARATIONS

Pre-Shave Talc Stick

A	VEEGUM	1.9
	Water	q.s.
B	Zinc stearate	4.7
	Light magnesium carbonate	1.9
	Talc	91.5
	Preservative	q.s.

Slowly add VEEGUM to the water, while agitating at maximum available shear. Continue mixing until smooth. Blend B. Add A to B and work into a smooth paste. Add more water as desired. Pack in stick mold and allow to dry.
Consistency: Rigid stick.
Suggested Packaging: Push or twist -up dispenser.

Shaving Cream

#1

Stearic Acid	6.00
Coco Fatty Acid	0.70
Triethanolamine	3.82
Propylene glycol	1.88
Glycerin	2.00
MACKAMIDE C	1.00
Sodium Lauryl Sulfate (30%)	2.50
Sorbitol 70%	1.88

Water Q.S. to	100.00
Fragrance	q.s.
MACKSTAT DM	q.s.

In maintank heat water add TEA, Propylene Glycol, glycerin, Sorbitol, heat to 75 degrees C. In separate vessel melt Stearic Acid, Coco Fatty Acid, Lanolin to 70 degrees C. add with mixing to maintank. Add Mackamide C mix 20 minutes cool and at 35 degrees C. add remainder.

Properties:	
pH	8.4-8.6
Fill Ration:	
Isobutane	3.47-3.5
Concentrate	96.5

#2

(Ladies)

A	VEEGUM	3
	Water	84
B	Glycerin	2
	Sorbitol 70%	3
	TRITON X-100	3
C	MYRJ 45	5
	Preservative	q.s.

Slowly add VEEGUM to the water, while agitating at maximum available shear. Continue mixing until smooth. Add B to A and heat to 70°C. Heat C to 75°C. Add C to A/B and mix until smooth and uniform.

Consistency: Soft cream.
Suggested Packaging: Jar or squeeze tube.

#3

(Aerosol)

Oil Phase	
GLUCAM E-20 Distearate	5.0
Stripped Coconut Fatty Acids	2.0
Stearic Acid, xxx	5.5

AMERLATE LFA	0.8
Lauramide DEA	0.5
Water Phase	
Carbomer 941 (3% aq.)	3.0
Deionized water	79.6
Triethanolamine (99%)	3.6
Perfume and preservative	q.s.

Heat the oil phase to 70°C. Heat water phase minus the triethanolamine to 70°C. Add water phase to oil phase at 70°C and immediately add the triethanolamine. Cool while mixing to 35°C and add the perfume.

Fill Procedure: 97% Concentrate: 3% Propellant A-46.

#4

(Aerosol)

Concentrate Phase	
GLUCQUAT 100	2.00
SOLULAN 25	1.50
SOLULAN 5	0.50
Stearic Acid, xxx	5.00
Triethanolamine (99%)	2.62
Deionized water	88.38
Perfume and preservative	q.s.

Concentrate Procedure: Combine deionized water, SOLULAN 25, SOLULAN 5, triethanolamine and preservative, and heat to 80-85°C with propeller agitation. Separately heat stearic acid and add to batch. Continue mixing at 80°C for fifteen minutes. Add GLUCQUAT 100 and cool to room temperature with mixing.

Aerosol Fill Procedure: Fill concentrate into shave cream cans and charge with A-46 hydrocarbon propellant using 92% concentrate and 8% propellant.

#5

(Ultra Aerosol for Sensitive Skin)

A	VEEGUM® Ultra	1.00
	Deionized Water	75.80
B	Glycerin	3.00
	Triethanolamine	4.00
C	Stearic Acid XXX	6.00
	Coconut Acid	1.30
	Mineral Oil	2.50
	Cetyl Alcohol	1.00
	VANOX PCX	0.20
D	VANSEAL NACS-30	5.00
	Methylparaben	0.20
	Fragrance	q.s.

Sift VEEGUM *Ultra* into the water while stirring with a propeller mixer at 700 rpm. Increase the mixer speed to 1700 rpm and mix for 30 minutes. Add the B ingredients in the order shown while mixing at 1700 rpm and heating to 75°C. Mix the C ingredients and heat to 75°C. slowly Add C to A and B. Adjust the mixer speed to avoid air entrapment and excessive foaming. Mix for 10 minutes at 75°C, then slow the mixer while cooling to 30°C. Add the D ingredients in the order shown and mix each until uniform. Package in aerosol containers using 95.0 wt. % of formula and 5.0 wt. % A-46 propellent.

Properties:
Viscosity - 500-700 cps
pH - 8.0 ± 0.2

#6

(Aerosol with Conditioner)

Concentrate Formula

Oil Phase

AMERLATE P	0.80
AMERLATE LFA	1.00

SOLULAN 98	1.00
Stearic Acid, xxx	4.00
Lauramide DEA	0.50
Water Phase	
POLYOX WSR N-750	15.00
QUATRISOFT POLYMER LM-200	25.00
GLUCAM E-20	2.00
Triethanolamine	2.58
Deionized water	48.12
Perfume and preservative	q.s.

Prepare aqueous solution of POLYOX WSR N-750 by sprinkling in room temperature water with adequate propeller agitation. Mix until uniform. Prepare QUATRISOFT Polymer LM-200 aqueous solution by sprinkling in room temperature water with propeller agitation. When well dispersed, heat to 75-80°C to accelerate hydration. Mix until clear and uniform. Heat both polymer solutions to 85°C. Add polymer solutions to 85°C water. When uniform, add remainder of water phase. Maintain at 85°C. Heat oil phase to 85°C. When uniform add to water phase. Mix while cooling to room temperature with adequate agitation. Package in aerosol can and charge with propellant.

Fill Procedure: 92% Concentrate: 8% Propellant A-46.

Shaving Gel

#1

Water	q.s
CELLOSIZE® Polymer PCG-10	1.25
POLYOX® WSR-205	0.10
Water	3.23
Palmitic Acid	6.00
Triethanolamine (99%)	5.00
AMEROXOL® OE-20	2.00
Glycerin	2.00
Isopentane	6.00
Fragrance, Preservative, Color	q.s.

Add CELLOSIZE® Polymer PCG-10 to water at room temperature with rapid stirring. When well dispersed heat to 75°C. Make a 3% solution using 0.1% of POLYOX® added to 3.23% water. Add to the CELLOSIZE® dispersion as it is heating to 75°C. When the batch is 75°C and a clear gel has formed, add Palmitic Acid, Triethanolamine, AMEROXOL® OE-20, Glycerin and the Preservative system to the batch individually waiting for each ingredient to dissolve before adding the next one. When the batch is uniform, cool to room temperature and add Fragrance and Color. Allow air to escape from the mixture. Cool Isopentane and shave gel to 15°C. Add isopentane slowly to batch with gentle stirring to avoid introducing foam. Package in sepro-type aerosol cans with A-40 propeelant.

#2

(Emulsifier-free)

A	VEEGUM	5.0
	Water	82.0
B	AMERCHOL L-101	2.5
	ACETULAN	0.5
	DOW CORNING[41] 200 Fluid (350 cs)	10.0
	Preservative	q.s.

Slowly add VEEGUM to the water, while agitating at maximum available shear. Continue mixing until smooth. Continue stirring, add B and mix until uniform.

Consistency: Thick cream.
Suggested Packaging: Jar or squeeze tube.

Aftershave

#1

(Conditioner)

Phase A:

CARBOPOL 934	0.4
Water	66.7
GLUCAM® E-20	4.3

Phase B:	
AMERLATE® P	2.0
PROPAL	1.5
MODULAN®	0.5
OHlan®	0.5
SOLULAN® 16	1.0
PROMULGEN® D	2.5
Phase C:	
Triethanolamine, 10% in water	4.0
Phase D:	
Menthol crystals	0.1
Perfume oil	1.5
Specially Denatured Alcohol No. 40	15.0
Preservative	q.s.

Phase A: Disperse Carbopol 934 thoroughly in water at 80°C; add Glucam E-20. Phase B: Heat all ingredients to 80°C. Add Phase A to Phase B with good stirring. Continue stirring to 50°C, add Phase C, triethanolamine. At 45°C slowly add premixed Phase D with good stirring. Stir with cooling to 30°C.

For greater fragrance duration and emollience, add Glucam P-20 to Phase A. For greater stimulation, increase alcohol concentration.

#2

(Stimulating, Cooling)

Perfume oil	0.7
Specially Denatured Alcohol No. 40	60.0
GLUCAM® E-10	4.0
GLUCAM® P-20	3.0
Water	32.3
Color	q.s.

Dissolve the perfume oil in the alcohol and add each ingredient in the order listed, stirring thoroughly after each addition. Age, chill and filter.

For added stimulation and cooling, add 0.1% menthol. To add astringent properties, add small amount of aluminum chlorhydrate solution.

#3

(Clear Viscous)

Phase A:	
Water	42.2
CARBOPOL 941	1.0
GLUCAM® P-20	5.0
Phase B:	
SOLULAN® 98	3.0
Specially Denatured Alcohol No. 40	45.0
Perfume oil	0.8
Phase C:	
Triethanolamine 10% in water	3.0

Phase A: Disperse Carbopol 941 thoroughly with good mixing at 60°C. Add Glucam P-20. Phase B: Dissolve Solulan 98 in alcohol with mixing and slight warming. Add perfume oil while stirring. Add Phase B to Phase A at 45-50°C in thin stream with good stirring. When homogeneous, add Phase C triethanolamine solution while stirring. Stir to 30°C.

To opacify, add small amount of Glucate SS to Phase B. For greater slip, replace part of Carbopol 941 with Polyox WSR N-80.

#4

(Stimulating, Fragrant)

Phase A:	
SOLULAN® C-24	3.0
SOLULAN® L-575	5.0
Water	9.6
GLUCAM® E-10	2.5
GLUCAM® P-20	3.0
Allantoin	0.2
Panthenol	0.2
Lemon juice, clarified	30.0
Witch Hazel	12.5
Phase B:	
Perfume oil	1.5

GLUCAMATE® SSE-20	2.5
Specially Denatured Alcohol No. 40	30.0
Color and preservative	q.s.

Phase A: Warm Solulans C-24 and L-575 together until liquid, mix with all other ingredients of Phase A. Phase B: Warm perfume oil and Glucamate SSE-20 until liquid and dissolve in alcohol. Add Phase B to Phase A with good stirring until homogeneous. Allow to stand overnight and filter to clarity. Lemon juice can be replaced by citric acid solution.

#5

(Moisturizing)

A	VEEGUM	1.0
	Water	80.4
B	SIPON LSB	3.4
	Glycerin	2.0
	Allantoin	0.1
C	CARBOWAX 400	4.0
	Isopropyl myristate	1.0
	ACETULAN	2.0
	Lecithin	1.0
D	SD Alcohol 40	5.0
	Menthol	0.1
	Preservative	q.s.

Slowly add VEEGUM to the water, while agitating at maximum available shear. Continue mixing until smooth. Add B to A and heat to 70°C. Heat C to 75°C. Add C to A/B with mixing to 40°C. Add D and mix until cool and uniform.

Consistency: Pourable lotion.
Suggested Packaging: Bottle.

#6
(Non-tacky)

A	VEEGUM	1.5
	Water	39.1
	DOW CORNING FG-10 Antifoam	0.2
B	DOW CORNING[41] 200 Fluid (350 cs)	3.0
	TWEEN 60	3.0
	AMERCHOL L-101	1.5
C	Klucel GF	1.5
	SD Alcohol 40	30.0
	Menthol USP	0.2
	Water	20.0
	Preservative	q.s.

Slowly add VEEGUM to the water, while agitating at maximum available shear. Continue mixing until smooth. Add antifoam. Blend B ingredients well. Add B to A while mixing. Prepare C by first dissolving menthol in alcohol and water. Slowly add Klucel GF, mixing until dissolved. Add C to A/B and mix until emulsion is uniform.

Consistency: Flowable lotion.
Suggested Packaging: Squeeze bottle.

AFTER SHAVE SOOTHER

Phase A

KYTAMER™ PC	0.5
Deionized Water	54.5

Phase B

GLUCAM® P-20	5.0
SD Alcohol 40 (Anhydrous)	40.0
Perfume and Preservative	q.s.

Disperse KYTAMER™ PC in water at room temperature using high speed agitation. When completely dispersed begin heating to 75°C with mixing.

Mix at 75°C until clear. Allow solution to cool to room temperature. Dissolve GLUCAM® P-20, perfume and preservative in the SD Alcohol 40 at room temperature. Mix until clear. Slowly add to the KYTAMER™ PC aqueous solution at room temperature and mix until clear and uniform.

SKIN CONDITIONING AFTER-SHAVE BALM

Phase A	
QUATRISOFT Polymer LM-200	0.5
Water	19.5
Phase B	
Carbomer 934	0.2
Water	56.8
Phase C	
GLUCAM E-20 Distearate	2.0
PROMULGEN D	2.5
PROPAL	1.5
Triethanolamine (10% aq.)	2.0
Phase D	
SD Alcohol 40	15.0
Perfume	q.s.

Add QUATRISOFT Polymer LM-200 to water (phase A) at room temperature until thoroughly dispersed and then heat to 45°C until completely hydrated. Prepare carbomer 934 solution (phase B). Add phase A to phase B with mixing while heating to 75°C. Heat phase C, minus the triethanolamine, to 75°C. Add AB to phase C at 75°C and mix while cooling to 50°C at which point add the triethanolamine. At 40°C add phase D. Mix and cool to 30°C and pour.

Chapter X

Sunscreen/Tan Products

Sunscreen Cream (W/O)

#1

I	APIFAC®	12.00
	Mineral Oil	10.00
	BEESWAX	1.00
	M.O.D.	6.00
	VEGETOL ® HUILEUX CALENDULA WL 1072	5.00
	PARSOL ® MCX	6.00
	Antioxygen	q.s.
	Preservative	q.s.
II	Demineralized Water	53.80
	CARBOPOL ® .934	0.30
	Glycerin	5.00
	Triethanolamine 99% (50% Sol.)	0.60
	Preservative	q.s.
	Perfume	0.30

Disperse the CARBOPOL ® . Let stand. Under stirring, pour II heated up to 80°C into I heated up to 80°C. Add the T.E.A. solution. Stir with a high speed stirrer for 2-3 mn. Cool down with moderate stirring. Around 35°C, add the other components.

#2

I	HYDROLACTOL ® .70	8.00
	Cetylacohol	1.00
	Mineral Oil	6.00

	VEGETOL ® HUILEUX CALENDULA WL 1072	3.00
	PARSOL ® MCX	7.50
	EUSOLEX ® 4360	2.00
	Antioxygen	q.s.
II	Demineralized Water	67.95
	Glycerin	3.00
	E.D.T.A. Tetrasodium Salt	0.05
	CARBOPOL ® .941	0.10
	Triethanolamine 99% (50% Sol.)	0.20
	CEVENYL ®	1.00
	Preservative	q.s.
	Perfume	0.20

Disperse the CARBOPOL ®. Let stand. Under moderate stirring, pour II heated up to 75°C into I heated up to 75°C. Add the T.E.A. solution and the CEVENYL ®. Cool down while stirring and around 30-35°C, add the other components.

#3
(Non-ionic, glossy)

Oil Phase

AMERSCREEN® P	3.0
PPG-3 Myristyl Ether	5.0
OHlan®	3.0
GLUCATE® SS	4.1
AMERCHOL L101®	5.0
Glyceryl Stearate and PEG-100 Stearate	5.0
Coconut Oil	5.0

Water Phase

GLUCAM® E-20	2.5
GLUCAMATE® SSE-20	0.9
Water	66.5
Perfume and Preservative	q.s.

Heat the oil and water phases to 80°C. Add water phase to the oil phase with stirring. Mix while cooling to 45°C, add perfume. Continue to cool while mixing and pack at 32°

SUNSCREEN LOTION

#1

(With Cocoa Butter O/W)

Oil Phase	
GLUCATE® DO	1.0
AMERSCREEN® P	2.0
Stearic Acid	3.0
Mineral Oil	5.0
Cocoa Butter	1.0
PPG-3 Myristyl Ether	3.0
Glyceryl Stearate	1.0
Water Phase	
Carbomer 934	0.3
Water	71.7
Triethanolamine (10% aq.)	12.0
Perfume & Preservative	q.s.

Heat the water to 75°C and disperse the Carbomer 934 with vigorous agitation. Heat the oil phase to 75°C and add the water phase to it with good agitation. Immediately add triethanolamine. Mix while cooling to room temperature. Add perfume below 40°C.

#2

(Ultra Violet Absorbing)

A	VEEGUM® *Ultra*	1.50
	Deionized Water	70.50
	Glycerin	5.50
B	PEG-150 Distearate	3.00
	Dioctyl Malate	2.00
	Mineral Oil	4.00
	Cetyl alcohol	0.50
	Benzophenone-3	3.00
	Octyl Dimethyl PABA	7.00
	Steareth-2	0.90
	Steareth-20	2.10
C	Preservative, Fragrance	q.s.

Heat the water to 55°C. Slowly add VEEGUM *Ultra* to the water while stirring with a propeller mixer at 500 rpm. Increase the mixer speed to 1500-1700 rpm and mix for 30 minutes, maintaining temperature at 55°C. Add glycerin and mix for 5 minutes. Mix B ingredients and heat to 60°C. Add B to A while mixing at 1500-1700 rpm. Continue mixing for 30 minutes. Avoid air entrapment. Slow mixing speed to 1000 rpm and continue mixing while cooling to 35°C. Add C and mix until uniform. Package.

Viscosity	5500cps***
pH	5.0

***Measured after 28 days aging at room temperature using Brookfield Viscometer, Model LV Spindle #4 at 60 rpm.

#3

A	VEEGUM	0.60
	RHODIGEL 23	0.15
	Water	65.45
	UNIMULSE CG	0.80
	Propylene glycol	3.00
B	FINSOLV TN	8.00
	UVINOL M-40	5.00
	PARSOL MCX	7.50
	RITACHOL	4.00
	TWEEN 80	0.50
C	Zinc oxide	5.00
	Preservative	q.s.

Blend VEEGUM and Rhodigel. Slowly add to the water, while agitating at maximum available shear. Continue mixing until smooth. Add remaining A ingredients slowly in order, mixing after each until uniform. Mix B well until the Uvinul M-40 dissolves. Add B to A and mix until smooth. Add C and mix until smooth and uniform.

Consistency: Pourable lotion.
Suggested Packaging: Opaque squeeze container.

#4
(Non-oily)

Part I	
Water	76.5
MONAQUAT P-TS	3.0
Sorbitol (70%)	5.0
Part II	
Glyceryl Stearate	3.0
Dimethicone and Trimethysiloxysilicate	3.0
Myristyl Myristate	1.0
Octyldimethyl PABA	5.0
Benzophenone-3	3.0
Tocopheryl Acetate	0.5

Heat Part I to 65°C with stirring. Heat Part II to 65°C with stirring. Add Part II to Part I with agitation. Stir while cooling to 40°C. Add fragrance, coloring, or preservative as required and package while warm.

#5
(Medium Viscosity)

A	VEEGUM	1.00
	RHODIGEL	0.20
	Glycerin	5.50
	Deionized Water	68.80
B	A-C 617G Polyethylene	2.00
	Glyceryl Monostearate, SE	3.00
	Dioctyl Malate	2.00
	Cetyl Alcohol	0.50
	Mineral Oil	4.00
	Steareth-2	0.30
	Steareth-20	2.70
	Benzophenone-3	3.00
	Octyl Dimethyl PABA	7.00
C	Preservative, Fragrance	q.s.

Dry blend VEEGUM and RHODIGEL. Add VEEGUM/RHODIGEL blend to water preheated to 85-90°C. Hydrate using maximum available shear until smooth, uniform and free of undispersed particles. Add glycerin and maintain temperature at 85-90°C. In a separate container, add all B ingredients and heat to 85-90°C until all components are in a liquid state. Stir gently as necessary. Slowly add B to A and homogenize for 5 minutes. Cool emulsion quickly to room temperature with gentle stirring. Add C and mix until uniform.

Consistency: Flowable Liquid; Viscosity measured after 30 days at room temperature: 1500-1900 cps using Brookfield Model LV, Spindle 4 at 60 rpm. Ph: 6.8-7.2.

Suggested Packaging: Plastic bottles or tubes.

#6

(Medium Viscosity)

A	VEEGUM	1.00
	RHODICEL	0.20
	Glycerin	5.50
	Deionized Water	70.80
B	Glyceryl Monostearate, SE	3.00
	Dioctyl Malate	2.00
	Cetyl Alcohol	0.50
	Mineral Oil	4.00
	Steareth-2	0.30
	Steareth-20	2.70
	Benzophenone-3	3.00
C	Preservative, Fragrance	q.s.

Dry blend VEEGUM and RHODIGEL. Add VEEGUM/RHODIGEL blend to water preheated to 75 to 85°C. Hydrate using maximum available shear until smooth, uniform and free of undispersed particles. Add glycerin and maintain temperature at 75 to 85°C. In separate container, add all B ingredients and heat to 75 to 85°C until all components are in a liquid state. Stir gently as necessary. Slowly add B to A and homogenize for 5 minutes.

Cool emulsion to room temperature with gentle stirring. Add C and mix until uniform.

Consistency: Flowable liquid; viscosity measured after 30 days at room temperature: 750 to 1000 cps using Brookfield Model LV, Spindle 4 to 60 rpm. pH: 6.8 to 7.2..

#7

A	VEEGUM	0.60
	RHODIGEL 23	0.15
	Water	65.45
	UNIMULSE CG	0.80
	Propylene glycol	3.00
B	FINSOLV TN	8.00
	UVINUL M-40	5.00
	PARSOL MCX	7.50
	Ritachol	4.00
	TWEEN 80	0.50
C	Zinc Oxide	5.00
	Preservative	q.s.

Add the VEEGUM/Rhodigel dry blend to the water slowly, agitating at maximum available shear until smooth. Add the remaining A ingredients in order, mixing after each until smooth and uniform. Mix B well until the Uvinul dissolves. Add B to A and mix until smooth. Add C and mix until smooth and uniform.

Sunscreen Oil

I	Coconut Oil	10.00
	LABRAFIL ® ISOSTEARIQUE	20.00
	VEGETOL ® HUILEUX CALENDULA WL 1072	15.00
	PARSOL ® MCX	4.00
	Mineral Oil	50.50
	Antioxygen	q.s.
	Perfume	0.50

Heat I up to 40°C until coconut oil is melted. Then add the other components.

Sun Screen Stick

#1

ROSS WHITE BLEACHED BEESWAX	20.0
ROSS PURE REFINED CANDELILLA WAX	16.1
ROSS PURE #1 YELLOW CARNAUBA WAX	4.0
Petrolatum	16.1
IPM	10.0
Mineral Oil 60/70	32.6
ROSS JOJOBA OIL	1.2
AMERSCREEN P	q.s.

Heat all ingredients is a steam jacketed kettle to 170 F under agitation. When fully mixed cool to 145 F and package. (Note: Capping may be necessary).

#2

I	BASE POUR STICK PL 1916	84.70
	PARSOL® MCX	8.00
	EUSOLEX® 4360	2.00
II	TIMIRON ® SUPERSILK MP 1005	2.00
	LABRAFIL ® ISOTEARIQUE	3.00
	Perfume	0.30

Heat I up to 80°C. Prepare II by mixing carefully until complete homogenization. Pour II into I. Add perfume. Around 65-70°C, pour into molds.

Solar Tanning Cream

#1

(Super Protection)

Part (A)

Water	69.1
Carbomer 934	.6

Part (B)

PROTOX T 25	.2
ROSSWAX 573	.8
ROSSWAX 1824	2.4
ROSS JOJOBA OIL	1.0
GMS-SE	.8
COCONUT OIL #76	3.2
ESCOLAL 507	8.0
ESCOLAL 567	4.5
ESCOLAL 557	7.5

Part (C)

GERMABEN II	1.0

Part (D)

Fragrance	q.s.

Part (E)

Triethanolamine	0.9

Heat the waxes in a steam jacketed kettle and add the Carbomer 934 under agitation. Heat Part (B) in a steam jacketed kettle until clear under agitation. When fully mixed add Part (B) to Part (A) under agitation.Then add Part (C) and mix thoroughly. Next add Part (D) and finally add Part (E) with agitation. Cool to 120. F and package.

#2

(High Protection)

Part (A)

Water	79.9
Carbomer 934	.6

Part (B)

PROTOX T 25	.2
ROSSWAX 573	.8
ROSSWAX 1824	2.0
ROSS JOJOBA OIL	.8
GMS-SE	.8

COCONUT OIL #76	3.0
ESCOLAL 507	7.0
ESCOLAL 567	3.0

Part (C)

GERMABEN II	1.0

Part (D)

Fragrance	q.s.

Part (E)

Triethanolamine	0.9

Heat the water in a steam jacketed kettle and add the Carbomer 934 under agitation. Heat Part (B) in a steam jacketed kettle until clear under agitation. When fully mixed add Part (B) to Part (A) under agitation. Then add Part (C) and mix thoroughly. Next add Part (D) and finally add Part (E) with agitation. Cool to 120. F and package.

#3

Water Phase:

Water	410.0
Carbomer 934	3.0

Oil Phase:

PROTOX T-25	1.0
ROSSWAX 573	4.0
GMS SE	4.0
COCONUT OIL #76	16.0
Jojoba Oil	4.0
ROSSWAX 1824	12.0
ESCALOL 507	25.0
Fragrance	q.s.
GERMABEN II	4.8
Triethanolamine	4.4

Disperse the Carbomer 934 in the water. In a second vessel heat the Oil Phase including the Escalol 507 until completely clear. When both phases are ready add the Oil Phase to the Water Phase. Add the preservative,

Fragrance and add the Triethanolamine under high agitation. When fully mixed you may package.

#4

Water Phase:	
Water	427.9
Carbomer 934	3.0
Oil Phase:	
PROTOX T-25	1.0
ROSSWAX 573	4.0
GMS SE	4.0
COCONUT OIL #76	16.0
Jojoba Oil	4.0
ROSSWAX 1824	12.0
ESCALOL 507	25.0
Fragrance	q.s.
GERMABEN II	5.0
Triethanolamine	4.4

Disperse the Carbomer 934 in the water. In a second vessel heat the Oil Phase including the Escalol 507 until completely clear. When both phases are ready add the Oil Phase to the Water Phase, add the Preservative, fragrance and add the Triethanolamine under high agitation. When fully mixed you may package.

Water Resistant Suntan Cream & Lotion

		Cream	Lotion
A	VEEGUM	2.0	1.75
	Water	69.5	75.50
	Glycerin	3.5	2.25
B	AMERSCREEN P	2.0	2.00
	ARLACEL 20	3.5	3.50
	TWEEN 20	4.5	4.50
	Dow Corning 556 Fluid	5.0	5.00
	Stearic acid xxx	5.0	5.50
	KESSCO GLYCEROL MONOSTEARATE S.E.	5.0	-

Preservative	q.s.	q.s.

Slowly add VEEGUM to the water, while agitating at maximum available shear. Continue mixing until smooth. Add the glycerin and mix until uniform. Heat A to 70°C. Heat B to 75°C. Add B to A, mixing until cool.

Consistency: Medium viscosity cream; Medium viscosity lotion.
Suggested Packaging: Cream Opaque tube; Lotion Opaque squeeze or pump bottle.

Suntan Lotion

(Extra Rich)

A	VEEGUM	1.0
	Water	86.0
	Propylene glycol	3.0
B	Stearic acid xxx	2.0
	DOW CORNING 556 FLUID	1.0
	Cetyl alcohol	0.5
	ACETULAN	4.0
	GIV-TAN F	2.0
	Triethanolamine	0.5
	Preservative	q.s.

Slowly add VEEGUM to the water, while agitating at maximum available shear. Continue mixing until smooth. Add the propylene glycol and mix until uniform. Heat A to 70°C. Heat B to 75°C. Add B to A, mixing until cool and uniform.
Consistency: Flowable lotion.
Suggested Packaging: Opaque squeeze or pump bottle.

Solar Tanning Lotions

Part I	#1	#2	#3	#4
Water	568.0	568.0	568.0	568.0
Carbomer 934	2.0	2.0	2.0	2.0

Part II				
ROSSWAX 573	4.0	4.0	4.0	4.0
GMS SE	4.0	4.0	4.0	4.0
Jojoba Oil	4.0	4.0	4.0	4.0
ESCALOL 507	13.0	19.0	25.0	32.0
Part III				
Fragrance	q.s.	q.s.	q.s	q.s.
Part IV				
GERMABEN II	6.0	6.0	6.0	6.0
Part V				
Triethanolamine	4.0	4.0	4.0	4.0

Heat the water with agitation and add the Carbomer 934. In a separate steam jacketed kettle melt Part II until clear. As soon as everything is melted add Part II to Part I with agitation. Then add Part III and Part IV with increased agitation: then add Triethanolamine. Cool to 130. F and package.

#5
(High Protection)

Water	517.0
Carbomer 934	1.8
ROSSWAX 573	2.0
GMS SE	3.6
Jojoba Oil	3.6
ESCALOL 507	42.0
ESCALOL 567	18.0
GERMABEN II	6.0
Fragrance	q.s.
Triethanolamine	3.6

Heat the water with agitation and add the Carbomer 934. In a separate steam jacketed kettle melt the oil phase till clear with agitation. Now add the oil phase to the water phase with agitation, add the Germaben II, fragrance and finally add the Triethanolamine with high agitation. Next cool to 130. F and package.

#6

(Super Protection)

Water	381.5
Carbomer 934	1.5
ROSSWAX 2540	3.0
GMS-SE	3.0
White Jojoba Oil	3.0
ESCALOL 507	40.0
ESCALOL 567	22.5
ESCALOL 557	37.5
GERMABEN II	5.0
Fragrance	q.s.
Triethanolamine	3.6

Heat the water in a steam jacketed kettle with agitation and add the Carbomer 934. In a separate steam jacketed kettle melt the oil phase until clear with agitation. Now add the oil phase to the water phase with agitation, then the Germaben II, then the Fragrance and finally add the Triethanolamine with high agitation. Next cool to 130.F and package.

Solar Tanning Oils

	#1	#2	#3	#4
COCONUT OIL #76	15.0	14.0	13.0	12.0
DOW CORNING #344	16.0	16.0	16.0	16.0
Isopropyl Myristate	13.0	13.0	13.0	13.0
Mineral Oil #7	42.0	42.0	42.0	42.0
ACETULAN	8.0	8.0	8.0	8.0
GLUCAM P-20	2.0	2.0	2.0	2.0
Jojoba Oil	2.0	2.0	2.0	2.0
ESCALOL 507	2.0	3.0	4.0	5.0
Fragrance	q.s.	q.s.	q.s.	q.s.

Mix all of the above ingredients in a stainless steel vessel, run thru a filter and package.

Solar Tanning Oil Mousse

Part (A)

ROSS BASE OIL 2539	62.3
ESCALOL 507	5.0
ARLACEL 60	3.0

TWEEN 60	4.0

Part (B)

Water	24.7
GERMABEN II	1.0
Fragrance	q.s.

Heat Part (A) and Part (B) in separate stainless steel vessels under gentle agitation to 170. F. When temperature is reached and both are clear, add Part (B) to Part (A) cool to 120. F. Fragrance and package.

Aerosol Fill:
90% of above concentrate
10% of A-46 Propellent
Note: Pack in Epon lined cans with Precision Valve Systems.

Water-in-oil Suntan Stick

A	VEEGUM	1.0
	Water	40.0
	Glycerin	3.0
B	Mineral Oil	12.5
	ACETULAN	5.0
	DOW CORNING 200 FLUID (350cs)	5.0
	Petrolatum	4.0
	Paraffin	20.0
	Stearic acid xxx	4.0
	GIV-TAN F	2.0
	PATIONIC CSL	3.0
	WITCAMIDE 511C	0.5
	Preservative	q.s.

Slowly add VEEGUM to the water, while agitating at maximum available shear. Continue mixing until smooth. Add glycerin and heat to 85-90°C. Heat B with stirring to 85-90°C. Add A to B and mix until smooth. Pour into molds and cool.
Consistency: Firm stick.
Suggested Packaging: Opaque push or twist action dispenser.

Solar Tanning Stick

#1
(White Color)

ROSSWAX 26-1152	15.0
ROSSWAX 1641	15.0
ROSSWAX 1824	20.0
Mineral Oil	17.5
DOW SILICONE 344	8.0
Isopropyl Myristate	6.5
COCONUT OIL #76	5.0
ACETULAN	4.0
GLUCAM P-20	2.0
Jojoba Oil	2.0
ESCALOL 507	5.0
Fragrance	q.s.
Preservative	q.s.

Load the waxes and the oils in a steam jacketed kettle, under agitation until melted. Cool to just before cloudy, add preservatives. Mold in containers. (Note: Capping may be necessary).

#2
(Tan Color)

ROSSWAX 26-1152	30.0
ROSSWAX 1824	20.0
Mineral Oil #7	17.5
DOW SILICONE 344	8.0
Isopropyl Myristate	6.5
COCONUT OIL #76	5.0
ACETULAN	4.0
GLUCAM P-20	2.0
Jojoba Oil	2.0
ESCALOL 507	5.0
Fragrance	q.s.
Preservative	q.s.

Heat the waxes and the oil in a steam jacketed kettle, to 175.F under agitation. When mixed fully, cool to just before cloudy, and add Fragrance and Preservative. Mold in containers. (Note: Capping may be necessary).

Tanning Jelly

Petrolatum USP	49.0
Mineral Oil #7	20.0
HENKEL CUTINA-LM	23.9
ROSS JOJOBA OIL	2.0
ESCALOL 507	5.0
Propyl Paraben	0.1
Fragrance	q.s.

Load ingredients in steam jacketed kettle and melt to a liquid state under agitation. When throughly mixed, cool to 130. F. Fragrance and package.

Tanning Accelerator

Part A	
Water	500.0
Carbomer 934	2.0
Part B	
ROSSWAX 1824	15.0
ROSSWAX 2540	6.0
GMS-SE	6.0
ROSS JOJOBA OIL	4.0
ESCALOL 507	12.0
COCONUT OIL #76	25.0
UNIPERTAN P-24	3.0
Part C	
GERMABEN II	6.0
Part D	
Fragrance	q.s.
Part E	
Triethanolamine	4.5

In a steam jacketed kettle heat the water and add the Carbomer 934 until fully dispersed under agitation. In a separate steam jacketed kettle melt the Oil Phase. When fully melted, add the Oil Phase to the Water Phase under agitation. Then add the Germaben II, then the fragrance and finally add the TEA with high agitation, until smooth. Cool to 130. F and package.

After Sun Care Lotion

I	TEFOSE® .1500	7.00
	Cetylacohol	1.00
	Sweet Almonds Oil	4.00
	VEGETOL ® HUILEUX CALENDULA WL 1072	2.00
	Antioxygen	q.s.
II	Demineralized Water	79.40
	Allantoin	0.10
	CARBOPOL ® .941	0.10
III	Triethanolamine 99% (50% Sol.)	0.20
	Demineralized Water	5.00
	PANCOGENE® .S	1.00
	Preservative	q.s.
	Perfume	0.20

Disperse the CARBOPOL ®. Let stand. Under moderate agitation, pour II heated up to 75°C into I heated up to 75°C. Add the triethanolamine solution. Cool down while stirring and around 30°C add III and the other components.

Chapter XI

Baby Products

Mild Baby Bubble Bath

MONATERIC 951A	30.0
MONATERIC LMAB	25.0
MONAMATE LNT-40	30.0
Preservative	0.3
Water	14.7

Combine ingredients. Adjust pH to 6.0 - 6.5.

Properties:

Appearance	Clear liquid
Nominal Activity	27%
Viscosity	500 cps

Baby Shampoo

#1

	Weight	Active
Water, Preservative	74.1	-
Alpha Olefin Sulfonate (40%)	9.6	3.9
MONATERIC LMM-30	12.8	3.8
Polysorbate 20	2.2	2.2
PEG-150 Distearate	1.3	1.3
	100.0	11.2

Add ingredients in order listed and blend while warming to 60°C.

pH = 6.8
Viscosity is approx. 2500 cps.

#2
(Ultra Mild)

	% Weight	% Active	% Solids
Water	50.2	-	-
Polysorbate 20	10.0	10.0	10.0
Methyl and Butyl Paraben	0.1	-	-
MONATERIC CSH-32	28.1	9.0	11.4
MONATERIC ISA-35	8.6	3.0	3.0
PEG-150 Distearate	3.0	3.0	3.0
	100.0	25.0	27.4

Add ingredients in the order listed and warm to 50°C with agitation before adding Monateric ISA-35 and PEG-150 distearate.

pH = 6.8 Viscosity is approximately 900 cps.

Baby Care Cream W/O

I	BASE MM 2007	18.00
	Mineral Oil	48.00
	PECEOL ® ISOSTEARIQUE	5.00
	Sweet Almonds Oil	2.00
	Preservative	q.s.
II	Demineralized Water	15.85
	Sodium Borate	0.85
	Zinc Oxyde	10.00
	Perfume	0.30

Pour II heated up to 90°C into I heated up to 90°C. Add the zinc oxyde while stirring, maintain up to 90°C for 2-3 mn. Stir with high speed stirrer for 2 mn. Cool down under moderate agitation. Add perfume. Homogenize if necessary.

Baby Lotion

#1

I	TEFOSE ® 1500	6.00
	PALMITATE DE CETYLE	2.00
	Sweet Almonds Oil	4.00
	Antioxygen	q.s.
II	Demineralized Water	85.50
	CARBOPOL ® 941	0.10
	Glycerin	2.00
	Triethanolamine 99% (50% Sol.)	0.20
	Perfume	0.20

Disperse the CARBOPOL ® . Let stand. Pour II heated up to 75°C into I heated up to 75°C. Add the triethanolamine solution. Cool down under moderate agitation. Add perfume.

#2
(Clear)

I	Demineralized Water	90.60
	Allanton	0.15
	VEGETOL ® HYDRO MATRICARE MCF 793	5.00
	Glycerin	3.00
	E.D.T.A. Tetrasodic Salt	0.05
	Dye C.I. 16255	q.s.
	Preservative	q.s.
	Perfume	0.30
	SOLUBILISANT GAMMA 2420	0.90

Mix all the components together in the order of formula. Mix the perfume and the SOLUBILISAT γ 2420 together. Filter.

Baby Wash

MACKADET BSC	15.0
MACKSTAT DM	q.s.
Water, Fragrance, Dye qs to	100.0

Add component to water and blend until clear.

Chapter XII

MISCELLANEOUS

Oil in Water Emulsion

	lbs.
MONAZOLINE O or T	8.20
Mineral oil	37.50
Glacial acetic acid	.75
Tall oil fatty acid	3.55
Water	50.00

Blend first four ingredients in order listed; mix until clear. Add blend to water slowly with continuous agitation. Note: the blend of the first four ingredients is useful as a corrosion-inhibiting coating oil which is completely water rinsable.

Water in Oil Emulsion

	lbs.
MONAZOLINE O or T	1.5
Mineral oil	25.0
Tall oil fatty acid	2.5
Water	71.0

Blend first three ingredients and follow with slow addition of water with continuous agitation. Further additions of water will increase the viscosity without causing emulsion phase inversion.

Fluid Emulsion

I	TEFOSE ® 2000	7.00
	Stearic Acid	1.00
	GELEOL ®	0.50

	Mineral Oil	3.00
	Apricot Kernel Oil	2.00
	Wheat Germ Oil	2.00
	D.P.P.G.	10.00
	Silicone 200 (100 CS)	2.00
	VEGETOL ® HUILEUX CALENDULA WL 1072	5.00
	D.L Alpha Tocopherol Acetate	0.05
	EUSOLEX 4360	0.50
	Antioxygen	q.s.
II	Demineralized Water	55.70
	CARBOPOL ® 941	0.15
	Propylene Glycol	5.00
	Triethanolamine 99% (50% Sol.)	0.30
	CEVENYL ®	0.50
	NUCLEODERM ® (2% Sol.)	5.00
	Preservative	q.s.
	Perfume	0.30

Disperse the CARBOPOL ®. Let stand. Under stirring pour II heated up to 75°C into I heated up to 75°C. Add the T.E.A. solution and the CEVENYL ®. Cool down while stirring and around 30-35°C, add the other components.

Bio Complex

I	Demineralized Water	69.60
	Glycerin	20.00
	CARBOPOL ® 941	0.10
	Sodium Hydroxyde (10% Sol.)	0.30
	Preservative	q.s.
	PHOSPHOSOMES ® CEVENYL 11.G	5.00
	PHOSPHOSOMES ® GINGKO BILOBA 15.G	5.00
	Perfume	q.s.
	Orange Dye	q.s.

Disperse the CARBOPOL ® in I. Let stand. Then add the other components in order of formula.

Dusting Powder

#1

Talc	97.7
Perfume oil	0.8
GLUCAM ® P-20	1.5
Preservative	q.s.

Premix a dry master batch of perfume oil, Glucam P-20 and 5% of the talc. Add master batch to remainder of talc. Mix until uniform.

For deodorant labeling, add sodium bicarbonate. To flesh-tint for aftershave, add iron oxide pigments.

#2

Talc	91.6
Magnesium carbonate	3.0
Zinc stearate	3.0
Triclosan	0.2
Perfume oil	0.7
GLUCAM ® P-20	1.5
Preservative	q.s.

Premix a dry master batch of Triclosan, perfume oil, Glucam P-20 and 5% of the talc. Mix with remaining talc and other ingredients until uniform.

For greater coverage, add zinc oxide or titanium dioxide. For light emollient effect, add Acetulan to the master batch mix.

Astringent Ointment W/O

Oil Phase:

OHlan™	7.5
Petrolatum, USP white	23.0
Mineral oil, 70 vis.	12.0
Silicone fluid 200, 350 cstks.	2.0
Ozokerite	3.5
Zinc oxide, U.S.P.	24.0

Water Phase:

Water	25.0
Sorbitol, 70% aq.	3.0
Perfume and Preservative	q.s.

Heat the oil phase (except zinc oxide) to 80°C to melt the ozokerite. Add the zinc oxide while mixing. Continue mixing until it is all wetted down and thoroughly dispersed. Add the water phase at 75°C to the oil phase at 75°C while mixing. Continue mixing while cooling to 45°C, add perfume. Stir to 35°C.

To impart elegance, replace petrolatum with AMERCHOL CAB. To reduce tackiness, replace Sorbitol with GLUCAM P-10. To improve lubricity, replace part of mineral oil with AMERLATE P.

Cream Depilatory

EVANOL	6.50
Calcium Thioglycolate	5.40
Calcium Hydroxide	7.00
Sodium Lauryl Sulfate	0.02
Sodium Silicate	3.43
Perfume	as desired
Water	q.s.

Heat the water to 75°C. Stirring, add the Lauryl sulfate, Sodium Silicate and Evanol. Continue stirring at 75°C until dissolved. Remove heat and continue stirring to room temperature. Add the Calcium Hydroxide and perfume. Finally, add the Calcium Thioglycolate powder to the cream. Continue stirring until uniform. Assay for Thioglycolic Acid content of 2.7%. Package.

Skin Bleach Cream

A	VEEGUM K	2.00
	Water	68.05
B	Glycerin	4.00
	Triethanolamine	1.00

C	Stearic acid xxx	2.00
	Cetyl alcohol	4.00
	Isopropyl myristate	2.00
	AMERCHOL L-101	10.00
	ARLACEL 165	3.00
D	Citric acid	0.30
	Hydroquinone	3.00
	Sodium sulfite	0.40
	Sodium metabisulfite	0.25
	Preservative	q.s.

Slowly add VEEGUM K to the water, while agitating at maximum available shear. Continue mixing until smooth. Add B to A and heat to 75°C. Heat C ingredients to 70°C and add to A/B with stirring. While stirring, cool to 65°C. Add the citric acid. Cool to 55°C. Add the hydroquinone. Cool to 45°C. Add the sodium sulfite, and then the sodium metabisulfite. Stir until cool and uniform.
Consistency: Soft Cream.
Suggested Packaging: Opaque jar.

Massage Oil

#1

SOLULAN P B 5	3.0
DOW CORNING SILICONE #344	16.0
EMEREST 2314	13.0
DRAKOL #9	31.0
Coconut Oil	31.0
ESCALOL 507	3.0
ROSS JOJOBA OIL	3.0
PERFUME NOVA ROME DE 51	q.s.

Load all ingredients into a vessel. Warm slightly until clear under agitation and package.

#2

(Jojoba)

Mineral Oil	61.5
Isopropyl Palmitate	24.0
Coconut Oil #76	5.0

Jojoba Oil	2.0
Almond Oil Sweet	2.0
ACETULAN	2.0
GLUCAM P-20	1.0
DOW CORNING SILICONE 344	2.0
Vitamine E	.5
Fragrance	q.s.

Load all ingredietns into a stainless steel kettle. Warm slightly until clear with agitation, add Fragrance and package.

Body Oil

Sun Flower Oil	3.00
LABRAFAC ® LIPO WL 1349	30.00
SILICONE FLUID 344	25.00
D.P.P.G.	38.50
38.50	
PARSOL ® MCX	3.00
Antioxygen	q.s.
Perfume	0.50

Mix all the components together.

Face Mask

(Oily)

#1

I	TEFOSE ® 2000	12.00
	GELEOL ®	2.00
	M.O.D. WL 2949	4.00
	VEGETOL ® HUILEUX CALENDULA WL 1072	3.00
	Antioxygen	q.s.
II	Demineralized Water	58.80
	Zinc Oxyde	10.00
	Kaolin	5.00
	Preservative	q.s.
	VEGETOL ® HYDRO BARDANE MCF 777	3.00
	ATELOGLYCANE ®	2.00
	Perfume	0.20

Disperse the powders in the water (part II). Under stirring pour II heated up to 75°C into I heated up to 75°C. Cool down while stirring and around 30°C, add the other components. Homogenize if necessary.

#2

(Creamy Clay)

A	VEEGUM	4.5
	RHODIGEL 23	0.2
	Water	73.8
	Glycerin	4.0
B	RITACHOL	4.5
	SYNCHROWAX BB4	1.0
	Cetyl alcohol	0.5
	CRODAMOL MM	1.5
	ARLACEL 40	0.5
	TWEEN 60	0.5
C	VANCLAY Kaolin	6.0
	Titanium dioxide	3.0
	Preservative	q.s.

Blend VEEGUM and Rhodigel. Slowly add the water, while agitating at maximum available shear. Continue mixing until smooth. Add glycerin and heat A to 70-75°C. Heat B to 70-75°C. Add A to B and mix until smooth. Add C. Mix until cool.
Consistency: Firm cream.
Suggested Packaging: Tube or cream jar.
Directions for Use:
Apply liberally to clean skin over face and throat. Allow to dry for 5 to 10 minutes. Rinse thoroughly with warm water and pat dry.

#3

(Peelable)

A	VEEGUM	1.5
	Water	58.5
	VINOL 523	10.0
	Propylene glycol	7.0

B	SD Alcohol 40	20.0
	HETOXOL OL-23	3.0
	Preservative	q.s.

Slowly add VEEGUM to the water, while agitating at maximum available shear. Continue mixing until smooth. Add propylene glycol with stirring and heat to 70-75°C. Slowly add Vinol 523, mixing until smooth and uniform. Continue mixing until 40°C. Dissolve Hetoxol Ol-23 in the alcohol. Add B to A and mix until smooth and uniform.
Consistency: Fluid lotion.
Suggested Packaging: Wide mouth jar with applicator brush.

The mask should be applied with a brush, spreading a thin uniform film on the skin. After approximately ten minutes, rinse or peel off.

Cuticle Softener Concentrate

NEODOL 25-3S	15.0
Sles (3 mole)	20.0
INCROMIDE LR	15.0
Propylene Glycol	10.0
INCRONAM BA-30	10.0
INCROMINE OXIDE BA	5.0
GERMABEN II	0.5
Deionized Water	17.5
KERASOL	
3.0	
Sodium Chloride	4.0

Combine all ingredients except Kerasol and sodium chloride. Mix until uniform, and add Kerasol. Then add sodium chloride with mixing. When all of the sodium chloride has dissolved, adjust the pH to 5.5 with citric acid (powder). Fill off.

Nail Polish Remover
(With conditioner)

Acetone	94.5
MACKALENE NLC	0.5
Deionized Water	5.0

Fragrance	q.s.

Add components together and blend until clear.

Mustache Wax

Lanolin USP	3.2
White USP Petrolatum	9.5
CERAPHYL 50S	31.6
CRYSTAL O	17.6
MINERAL OIL BLANDOL	6.3
ROSS OZOKERITE WAX 77W	6.3
CERAPHYL 41	9.4
ROSS WHITE BLEACHED BEESWAX	4.4
ROSS REFINED CANDELILLA WAX	4.4
ROSS REFINED #1 YELLOW	1.3
Carnauba Wax	
Preservative	6.0

Melt all ingredients in a steam jacketed kettle under agitation until clear. Cool to 130. F and package.

Pet Shampoo With Pyrethrin
#1

	% Weight	% Active
Water, preservative	59.6	-
Salt	0.1	-
SIPON ESY	32.0	8.0
MONATERIC CAB	5.0	1.5
MONAMID 1007	2.5	2.5
PYRENONE OT666**	0.8	0.1

Add first four ingredients and blend thoroughly. Dissolve Pyrenone in Monamid 1007 and add to the shampoo. Adjust pH to 6.0 - 7.0 range with phosphoric acid.

pH = 6.5 Viscosity is approx. 500 cps.

#2

	% Weight	% Active
Water	34.6	-
Magnesium Lauryl Sulfate (27.0%)	49.2	13.3
PYROCIDE INTERMEDIATE 5192	0.5	0.3
MONATERIC ISA-35	5.7	2.0
MONAMATE CPA-40	10.0	4.0
	100.0	19.6

Add first three ingredients and blend thoroughly while warming to 55°C. Add the last two components and stir with slow agitation. the pH must be increased to 6.5 to 7.0 with triethanolamine for the pyrocide to be effective.

pH = 6.5 Viscosity is approx. 1400 cps.

Deodorant Pet Shampoo With Coal Tar

	% Weight	% Active
Water, preservative	12.9	-
Ammonium Lauryl Sulfate (28.0%)	60.7	17.0
MONATERIC ISA-35	11.4	4.0
MONAMATE CPA-40	10.0	4.0
Coal Tar Extract (20%)	5.0	1.0
	100.0	26.0

Add the first four ingredients while warming to 40°C and stirring gently. When blended, remove heat and add the coal tar extract. Initially a haze may appear but it will gradually disappear.

pH = 6.0 Viscosity is approx. 1000 cps.

APPENDIX

Incompatible Chemicals

The substances in the left-hand column must be stored and handled so that they cannot come into any contact with the substances in the right-hand column.

Alkaline and alkaline-earth metals, such as sodium, potassium, cesium, lithium, magnesium, calcium, aluminum	Carbon dioxide, carbon tetrachloride, and other chlorinated hydrocarbons. (Also prohibit water, foam, and dry chemical on fires involving these metals.)
Acetic acid	Chromic acid, nitric acid, hydroxyl-containing compounds, ethylene glycol, perchloric acid, peroxides, and permanganates.
Acetone	Concentrated nitric and sulfuric acid mixtures.
Acetylene	Chlorine, bromine, copper, silver, fluorine, and mercury.
Ammonia (anhydr)	Mercury, chlorine, calcium hypochlorite, iodine, bromine, and hydrogen fluoride.
Ammonium nitrate	Acids, metal powders, flammable liquids, chlorates, nitrites, sulfur, finely divided organics or combustibles.
Aniline	Nitric acid, hydrogen peroxide.
Bromine	Ammonia, acetylene, butadiene, butane and other petroleum gases, sodium carbide, turpentine, benzene, and finely divided metals.
Calcium carbide	Water (See also acetylene.)
Calcium oxide	Water.
Carbon, activated	Calcium hypochlorite.
Copper	Acetylene, hydrogen peroxide.
Chlorates	Ammonium salts, acids, metal powders, sulfur, finely divided organics or combustibles.

Chromic acid	Acetic acid, naphthalene, camphor, glycerol, turpentine, alcohol, and other flammable liquids.
Chlorine	Ammonia, acetylene, butadiene, butane and other petroleum gases, hydrogen, sodium carbide, turpentine, benzene, and finely divided metals.
Chlorine dioxide	Ammonia, methane, phosphine, and hydrogen sulfide.
Fluorine	Isolate from everything.
Hydrocyanic acid	Nitric acid, alkalis.
Hydrogen peroxide	Copper, chromium, iron, most metals or their salts, any flammable liquid, combustible aniline, nitromethane.
Hydrofluoric acid, anhydrous (hydrogen fluoride)	Aqueous or anhydros ammonia
Hydrogen sulfide	Fuming nitric acid, oxidizing gases.
Hydrocarbons (benzene, butane, propane, gasoline, turpentine, etc.)	Fluorine, chlorine, bromine, chromic acid, sodium peroxide.
Iodine	Acetylene, anhydrous or aqueous ammonia.
Mercury	Acetylene, fulminic acid, ammonia.
Nitric Acid (conc)	Acetic acid, aniline, chromic acid, hydrocyanic acid, hydrogen sulfide, flammable liquids, flammable gases, and nitritable substances.
Nitroparaffins	Inorganic bases.
Oxygen	Oils, grease, hydrogen, flammable liquids, solids or gases.
Oxalic acid	Silver, mercury.
Perchloric acid	Acetic anhydride, bismuth and its alloys, alcohol, paper, wood, grease, oils.
Peroxides, organic	Organic or mineral acids; avoid friction.
Phosphorus (white)	Air, oxygen.
Potassium chlorate	Acids (See also chlorate.)
Potassium perchlorates	Acids (See also perchloric acid.)

Potassium permanganate	Glycerol, ethylene glycol, benzaldehyde, sulfuric acid.
Silver	Acetylene, oxalic acid, tartaric acid, fulminic acid, ammonium compounds.
Sodium	See alkaline metals.
Sodium nitrate	Ammonium nitrate and other ammonium salts.
Sodium oxide	Water.
Sodium peroxide	Any oxidizable substance, such as ethanol, methanol, glacial acetic acid, acetic anhydride, benzaldehyde, carbon disulfide, glycerol, ethylene glycol, ethyl acetate, methyl acetate, and furfural.
Sulfuric acid	Chlorates, perchlorates, permanganates.
Zirconium	Prohibit water, carbon tetrachloride, foam, and dry chemical on zirconium fires.

Safety in the Laboratory or Home Workshop

It is necessary to learn:

- Use of laboratory fume hoods
- Handling flammable solvents
- Mixing acids
- Glass blowing

- Common electrical hazards
- First aid (for four situations only)
  - Stoppage of breathing
  - Profuse bleeding
  - Chemical burns (water only)
  - Fire in clothing
- Use of portable fire extinguishers
- Compressed or flammable gases
- Disposal of hazardous chemicals
- Handling and storing dangerous chemicals, including alkali metals.

An outstanding deficiency pertaining to laboratory safety seems to be a lack of awareness of hazards among nontechnical personnel. It is conceivable that increased emphasis on "briefing" custodial workers about the dangers of the laboratories in which they work, and periodic review of these conditions could substantially reduce the hazard of ignorance.

Third, a more universal use of safety glasses, reaction shields, and other personal protective devices seems to be needed. From the responses received, an increased program of education on the hazards of common laboratory procedures and the use of personal protective equipment to lessen these hazards would be helpful.

Chemical Hazards

All laboratories, whether they be biological, chemical, or radiological, utilize hazardous chemicals. The hazard may result from utilizing the "raw" product or from products of a chemical reaction between two or more substances or breakdown products through heating or aging. Laboratory personnel should have an acquaintance at least with the modes of entry, the physiological responses, both acute and chronic, and methods of roughly assessing the hazards potential of chemicals they are using.

Electrical Hazards and Management

The problem of handling electricity is probably one of the most ignored facets of safety, yet each year many needless deaths and injuries are caused through carelessness in handling even low voltages. It is also of importance to recognize that electrical equipment can act as an ignition source to activate a fire or explosion. Static electricity should be considered in this category.

Pressure Hazards

Pressure equipment, either high or low (vacuum), is a part of most laboratories. High-pressure apparatus such as gas cylinders, if improperly handled, can be very dangerous. This is especially true of oxygen. Precautions are necessary in handling, transporting, and in storing. Vacuum equipment, through implosions, can be every bit as dangerous as high-pressure explosions.

Cryogenic Hazards

Cryogenics or the use of low-temperature refrigerants requires a knowledge of the behavior of these materials under laboratory conditions. It is impossible to understand the design of a piece of cryogenic equipment or cryogenic experiment without an appreciation for the principles of insulation or the significance of extremely low temperatures. Misuse can result in severe injury.

Flammable Chemicals-Hazards

Fires and explosions account for the most dangerous and the most expensive types of laboratory accidents. A knowledge of the flammable properties of chemicals along with an understanding of potential sources of ignition is extremely vital. Storage and handling of these materials also requires special attention.

General Safety Considerations

A number of accidents and injuries in laboratories could very well result from improper lifting, falls, and lacerations from improper handling of glassware. Preventive measures in these areas are worthy of mention.

Ventilation

The principal method of hazards control in laboratory involves the effective use of ventilation, both general and exhaust. An example of exhaust ventilation is the fume hood which if improperly designed or used fails to give the desired protection. Observations indicate that the function of this equipment is not entirely understood and a number of misuses have been witnessed.

Laboratory Sanitation

Poor laboratory sanitation practices may be the cause of contaminating potable water supplies through temporary cross connections. At times, poor housekeeping practices may be dangerous because of blocking passages or by providing tripping hazards. Many chemicals are kept well beyond their usefulness, causing containers to deteriote and leak, or chemicals to become unstable. Disposal of flammable and toxic chemicals also presents a problem.

Protective Equipment

All laboratories require that protective equipment of one type or another be immediately available. These devices may include eye wash, emergency shower, safety glasses, eye shields, protective clothing, and respiratory protection. Knowledge of the proper usage and limitations of such equipment is extremely important. At times, injury or death may result from improper selection and application of protective equipment.

Reports and Records

Reports and records are necessary adjuncts to any safety program and should be complete, accurate, and disseminated to the appropriate administrators. Accident reports are of little value unless periodically examined and tabulated in order to obtain a picture of local and overall problems.

Emergencies

The initial procedures one follows in an emergency oftentimes determine the ultimate outcome of the accident, both to the individuals and to the installation. The rudiments of first aid, fire fighting and reporting are vital. Personnel have to be continually instructed on procedures for medical and fire emergencies and how and where to make these initial contacts. Such procedures are critical, especially when working alone.

Contact Lenses

It is important to wear eye protection in the chemical laboratory and especially when wearing contact lenses.

Danger in Handling Acid

The heat evolution of the solution could have provided sufficient thermal shock to the glass to permit it to crack when lifted free of the counter, or setting it on a cold counter top; or a shock in setting it down, could have contributed to the bottom separating when the jug was lifted.

Written procedures for handling of acids should always be followed. Personal protective equipment consisting of face protection, rubber apron, and gloves are a necessity for this operation.

You Must Have Fire Extinguishers

If a fire breaks out in your office or apartment, get out fast. Many people are killed because they don't realize how fast a small fire can spread.

If you are caught in smoke take short breaths, breathe through your nose, and crawl to escape. The air is better near the floor.

Head for stairs - not elevator. A bad fire can cut off the power to elevators. Close all doors and windows behind you.

If you are trapped in a smoke-filled room, stay near the floor, where the air is better. If possible, sit by a window where you can call for help.

Feel every door with your hand. If it's hot don't open. If it's cool, make this test: open slowly and stay behind the door. If you feel heat or pressure coming through the open door, slam it shut.

If you can't get out, stay behind a closed door. Any door serves as a shield. Pick a room with a window. Open the window at the top and bottom. Heat and smoke will go out to the top. You can breathe out the bottom.

DON'T fight a fire yourself.

DON'T jump. Many people have jumped and died without realizing rescue was just a few minutes away.

If there is a panic for the main exit, get away from the mob. Try to find another way out. Once you are safely out, DON'T go back in. Call the Fire Department immediately. Use alarm box or telephone. DIAL 911.

If you find smoke in an open stairway or open hall, use another preplanned way out.

REMEMBER: Get out fast. Don't underestimate how fast a small fire can spread. Use stairs, not the elevator. Close all doors behind you. Don't panic. Once you are safely out, call the Fire Department. Dial 911 or use alarm box. don't go back in.

Where to Buy Materials

Some of the materials you need can be bought in your local drugstore. In some cases the druggist can order materials for you from suppliers. The yellow page section of the telephone book will contain a listing of local supply houses. If you are having difficulty obtaining a specific ingredient, check the Trademark Chemical Manufacturer's List in this Appendix. You can write directly to the company and ask them for a local supplier of their chemical.

Aerosols

The ISOTRON Department of the Pennwalt Corporation located in Philadelphia, Pennsylvania has been kind enough to supply the editors with the following information regarding the general preparation and use of aerosol products.

The functionality and popularity of the aerosol package has been proven by its high growth rate during the past twenty years. the appeal of this packaging technique has spread to practically every dispensable product that is conventionally sold in a small package. In addition, it has generated new products that are only possible in the aerosol form. Aerosols are found in such diverse fields as food, cosmetics, pharmaceuticals, household cleaners, insecticides and industrial lubricants.

The use of terms such as an aerosol chemist or aerosol chemistry has become popular in the past few years, however, they may be misleading to the extent that they imply expertise in the wide range of products involved in aerosol packaging. More properly an individual should be designated an aerosol paint chemist, an aerosol cosmetic chemist, etc. The transition of the cosmetic chemist to an aerosol cosmetic chemist involves gaining the experience and knowledge of propellent compatibility with cosmetics and how the ratio of propellent to product affects the dispensing variables (spray pattern, spray rate, etc.).The same transition can be made readily by chemists in other specialties.

There are, of course, formulating problems common to all aerosol products. These involve such things as spray pattern control, valve clogging, leakage and corrosion. Corrosion in an aerosol product is far more critical than in a conventional package, primarily because of safety considerations. An aerosol weakened by corrosion can explode and cause injuries or at least property damage. Even relatively small amounts of corrosion can cause problems such as valve clogging or color changes. Aerosol packages, due to their pressurized nature, are characterized as compressed gases by the U.S. Department of Transportation (D.O.T.). The D.O.T. has special regulations for aerosol packages which define the pressure limits, and package size and also specify the hot water test bath for almost all aerosol products. Formulators of aerosols should become familiar with these limitations.

General considerations when formulating a product for aerosol packaging should include the following:

1. *Desired Spray Pattern*

The ratio of propellent to product to a large extent controls the spray pattern achieved. In a system in which the propellent and product are miscible, propellent levels of 75% or more give a light dry spray such as in a room deodorant. At levels of 40% to 50%, a wet spray of the type found in paint sprays is the result. At 15% to 25% a stream is achieved. In nonmiscible systems (usually water containing products) the nature of the emitted product will depend largely on whether or not the system is in the form of an emulsion. Nonemulsified systems such as a starch need a mechanical break-up type valve to achieve a spray. Emulsified systems in which the water is the exterior phase usually form foams such as a shaving cream. Where the water is in the interior emulsion phase, nonfoaming sprays can be achieved.

2. *Viscosity Control*

In general the packaging of an aerosol means that the viscosity of the concentrate will have to be lower than a similar concentrate in conventional packages. In many cases a suitable diluent will have to be added or the solute changed to give a solution of the proper spray character.

3. *Solid Particles*

Formulations containing solid particles such as pigments, abrasives, cosmetic powders, etc., can cause problems in aerosols. The principle problem, of course, is due to the clogging of the valve by the particles. This may arise for several reasons:

a. Particals are too large. Obviously, if solid particles are in the same magnitude of size as the aerosol valve orifice, clogging of the valve can readily occur. As a rule of thumb, if the solid is screened through a 325 mesh screen, clogging for this reason will be minimal.

b. Particle agglomeration. Although the original particle size may be satisfactory, the formation of agglomerates in the aerosol may cause clogging. Maintaining contents of the solids at a low level and the addition of "dispersion aids" is helpful in minimizing this problem.

In addition to clogging, solid particles in an aerosol may cause other problems. Leakage of the valve after use is sometimes encountered. This is due to solid particles left on valve gasket surfaces which do not allow the valve to completely seal after use. Valve design and particle size control are important in minimizing this problem.

The low viscosity required for aerosol formulations means that settling of aerosol products is usually faster than with conventional packages.This fact, coupled with the unavailability of the aerosol product for redispersion means that often some of the solid particles are left in the container when the product is sprayed out. This can mean a loss of strength if the particle is an active material or a change in color value if pigments are involved. Glass marbles or steel balls are often included in the aerosol container to aid in redispersion but are not efficient in the bottom seam area.

A general practice in formulas containing solid particles is to use a shortened dip-tube so that the dip-tube will not extend into the settled layer. This minimizes the possibility of drawing up a "slug" of the settled material into the valve and causing clogging problems. Even though settled material on the bottom of the can might be adequately redispersed, such material in a dip-tube is not readily dispersed.

4. *Odors*

Difficulty may be encounter if the same perfume composition used in a conventionally packaged product is used in an aerosol package. Obviously the perfume may not be compatible with the propellent and other additives might be required to adapt the product to an aerosol. More subtly, however, the odor character of the perfume may change. This is due to the fact that the odor is being presented to the user in a different form; i.e. in a light spray instead of a liquid or as a liquid instead of a cream. Under these circumstances the most volatile perfume components are more quickly dissipated and some of the lesser volatile perfume materials are given enhanced volatility. In a light dry spray such as a room deodorant all the components are presented simultaneously to the user. Masking of the solvent and the slight propellent odor may also present a problem.

Most of the perfume supply houses have aerosol packaging facilities and are experienced in perfume formulation to deal with the problems noted above. It is suggested that aerosol formulators rely on them for assistance in this area.

5. *Choice of Valve and Actuator*

There are literally thousands of valve and button combinations available for use in aerosol products. The choice is narrowed down considerably when the formula composition is decided on and the approximate spray style is chosen. In order to make a good recommendation for valve and actuator the valve manufacturer needs to know the following:

a. Desired spray character

b. Flow rate

c. Composition of product (needed to determine appropriate gaskets and materials of construction)

6. *Choice of Container*

A wide variety of metal container sizes and materials of construction are available. Can suppliers are very helpful in suggesting the type of can needed depending on the chemical nature of the product. Glass bottles are useful for low pressure formulations where corrosion problems exist or there is a need for the aesthetic and purity character of glass.

Once the desired formulation has been chosen, it is necessary to begin to test the stability of the package. As noted previously, it is even more important in an aerosol package than conventional packages to eliminate corrosive tendencies and other formulation defects. In an aerosol package you do not have the luxury of being able to observe and to possibly correct product failures as you can with conventional packages.

Ideally a package should be shelf tested over the projected life of the package. Much information can be gained from accelerated test procedures however. Typically, accelerated tests are run by storing the package at temperatures of 130° F for a month or as low as 100° F for six months. The higher temperature gives more information on the corrosive nature of the product stability. During the shelf tests and the accelerated tests, samples should be examined periodically. Variables evaluated should include the following:

a. Weight loss

b. Appearance of corrosion

c. Valve functionality

d. Any changes in product efficacy, color or odor

Finally, once the formulation is perfected it will be necessary to design the appropriate label for the product making sure that the requirements of the various regulatory agencies have been met. Such agencies include the F.D.A., the U.S. Department of Agriculture, the New York City Fire Department and other local regulatory bodies.

Sample Label

(your brand name here)

Insect Repellent Lotion

Contains DEET* for longer protection - resistant to perspiration, water and wear. Not greasy.

Repels mosquitoes, biting flies, gnats, chiggers, ticks and fleas.

Active ingredient * N, N-diethyltoluamide	50%
*meta isomer	47.5%
*other isomers	2.5%
Inert ingredients	50%

Directions for Use: Shake into hands and rub lightly over all exposed skin, stockings and all other thin clothing. Reapply as necessary. For chiggers, ticks and fleas, use as above and also apply to socks, pant cuffs and around other openings in outer clothing. Safe to use on nylon, orlon, cotton and wool.

Caution: Harmful if swallowed. Avoid contact with eyes and lips. Keep out of reach of children.

Do not use on acetate, rayon and Dynel. May have plasticizing or softening action on certain synthetic fibers and paint and lacquer surfaces.

Manufactured by:

(customer's name
and address here) Net Weight Oz.

Trademark Chemicals

Trademark Chemical Suppliers

1. Air Products & Chemicals, Inc .... Allentown, Pa 18105
2. Akzo/Armak .... Chicago, IL 60606
3. Akzo Italia .... Milan, Italy
4. Alcolac Inc. .... Linthicum, MD 21090
5. Allied Signal .... Morristown, NJ 07960
6. Amerchol Corp/CPC Int' 1 Inc. .... Edison, NJ 08818
7. Amerchol Europe .... Vilvoorde, Belgium
8. Aqualon Co. .... Wilmington, DE 19850
9. Atlas Refinery Inc. .... Newark, NJ 07105
10. Atochem USA Inc. .... Paramus, NJ 07652
11. BASF Corp. .... Parsippany, NJ 07054
12. Cabot Corp. .... Tuscola, IL 61953
12a. CasChem Inc. .... Bayonne, NJ 07002
13. Ciba Geigy .... Greensboro, NC 27419
14. Croda Chemicals Ltd. .... N. Humberside, UK
15. Croda Inc. .... New York, NY 10010
16. Davison Chemical/W.R. Grace & Co. .... Baltimore, MD 21203
17. Dow Chemical Co. .... Midland, MI 48640
18. Dow Chemical Europe SA .... Horgen, Switzerland
19. Dow Corning Corp. .... Midland, MI 48640
20. Dragoco Corp. .... Totowa, NJ 07511
21. Exxon Co. USA .... Houston TX 77001
22. Ferro Corp .... Bedford, OH 44146
23. Fidco Inc. .... White Plains, NY
24. Finetex Inc. .... Elmwood Park, NJ 07407
25. GAF Corp. .... Wayne, NJ 07470
26. Gattefosse Corp. .... 69800 St. Priest, France
27. Givaudan Corp. .... Clifton, NJ 07014
28. Goldschmidt Chemical Corp. .... Hopewell, VA 23860
29. B.F. Goodrich & Co. .... Cleveland, OH 44131
30. W.R. Grace & Co. .... Lexington, MA 02173
31. A. Gross & Co. .... Newark, NJ 07101
32. Henkel Corp. .... Ambler, PA 19002
33. Henkel Canada .... Ville d'Anjou, PQ, Canada
34. Henkel/Emery Group .... Cincinnati, OH 45249
35. Hercules Inc. .... Wilmington, DE 19894
36. Heterene Chemical Co., Inc. .... Paterson, NJ 07513
37. Hoechst-Celanese Corp. .... Somerville, NJ 08876
38. ICI America Inc. .... Wilmington, DE 19897
39. ICI Specialty Chemicals .... Kortenberg, Belgium
40. Lipo Chemicals Inc. .... Paterson, NJ 07504
41. Lonza Inc. .... Fair Lawn, NJ 07410
42. McIntyre Chemical Co. Ltd. .... Chicago, IL 60632

43. McLaughlin Gormley King Co. .... Minneapolis, MN 55427
44. Mearl Corp. .... New York, NY 10017
45. Merck & Co. Inc. .... Rahway, NJ 07065
46. Millmaster-Onyx Int'l .... Fair Lawn, NJ 07007
47. Mona Industries Inc. .... Paterson, NJ 07544
48. National Starch & Chemical Corp. .... Bridewater, NJ 08807
49. New Jersey Zinc Co. .... Palmerton, PA 18071
49a. Nipon Oil & Fats Co. .... Tokyo, Japan
50. NL Treating Chemicals .... Houston, TX 77205
51. Olin Chemicals .... Stamford, CT. 06904
52. Penreco/Div. Pennzoil .... Butler, PA 16001
53. Petroleum Specialties Int'l/Croda .... New York, NY 10010
54. PPG Mazer .... Gurnee, IL 60031
55. Rhone-Poulenc Inc. .... Monmouth Junction, NJ 08852
56. RITA Corp. .... Crystal Lake, IL 60014
57. Robeco Chemicals Inc. .... New York, NY 10016
58. Rohm & Haas Co. .... Philadelphia, PA 19105
59. Rona Pearl/Div EM Industries .... Bayonne, NJ 07002
60. Frank B. Ross Co., Inc. .... Jersey City, NJ 07304
61. Shell Chemical Co. .... Houston, TX 77002
62. Stauffer Chemical Co. .... Westport, CT 06880
63. Stepan Co. .... Northfield, IL 60093
64. Sutton Laboratories Inc. .... Chatham, NJ 07928
65. Union Carbide .... Danbury, CT 06817
66. R.T. Vanderbilt & Co., Inc. .... Norwalk, Ct 06855
67. VanDyk & Co., Inc. .... Belleville, NJ 07109
68. Vista Chemical Co. .... Houston, TX 77224
69. Witco/Sonneborn .... New York, NY 10017

INDEX

D

E

F

H

L

M

N

O

P

R

S